Carlos Michel Albuquerque Peres
José Guilerme Caldas
Evandro Cesar Souza

Encephalic Arteriovenous Malformation

Carlos Michel Albuquerque Peres
José Guilerme Caldas
Evandro Cesar Souza

Encephalic Arteriovenous Malformation

Nidal architecture, embolization and radiosurgery

ScienciaScripts

This book is a translation from the original published under ISBN 978-620-2-04739-5.

Publisher:
Sciencia Scripts
is a trademark of
Dodo Books Indian Ocean Ltd. and OmniScriptum S.R.L publishing group

120 High Road, East Finchley, London, N2 9ED, United Kingdom
Str. Armeneasca 28/1, office 1, Chisinau MD-2012, Republic of Moldova, Europe
Managing Directors: Ieva Konstantinova, Victoria Ursu
info@omniscriptum.com

Printed at: see last page
ISBN: 978-620-2-73753-1

SUMMARY

With love, to my girlfriend and wife **Cristina**, an inseparable companion in my life since medical school. I admire her professional ability, preparation and total dedication to hematology patients. And my thanks for always stimulating and encouraging me to keep going.

To my son **Carlos Henrique** and my daughter **Raquel**, who have given meaning to my life. They are my greatest source of pride.

To my mother, **Glorinha**, my best Portuguese teacher (literally). My gratitude for her love and constant support.

To my father, **Carlos**, for his unconditional support for all my goals, always.

To my sisters, **Liége, Liana and Liliane**, all excellent professionals in their fields, for their encouragement and family support.

THANKS

To my advisor, **Prof. Dr. José Guilherme Mendes Pereira Caldas**, for his great teaching and methodological skills and for his always good-natured encouragement. I've learned a lot over the years, not just from this thesis, but from long discussions, from monitoring cases in hemodynamics and from the side projects we've developed. You can't stop the wind, but you can direct the sail so that the wind becomes favorable...

To **Dr. Evandro Cesar de Souza**, a tireless neurosurgeon rooted in radiosurgery, for allowing me to develop this work with the casuistry of patients treated at InRad.

To **Prof. Dr. Raymundo Soares de Azevedo Neto**, for his guidance on the correct analysis and statistical interpretation of the data I collected, as well as for the encouragement he gave me at a time when I didn't think I would continue.

To the members of the qualification committee, **Profs. Drs. Eberval Gadelha Figueiredo, Evandro Cesar de Souza and Eduardo Weltman**, for their pertinent and useful suggestions.

To the assistants, **Dr. Paulo Puglia Jr., Dr. Michel Eli Frudit and Prof. Dr. José Guilherme Mendes Pereira Caldas**, and to the residents of the Interventional Neuroradiology Service at InRad, who led the embolized patients, who helped me interpret the images and find clinical data for this study.

To the **nursing teams** and the secretary of the Interventional Radiology service at InRad, **Rosana Lopes**, for their help in finding "lost patients" in this study.

To Mrs. **Lia Melo**, the Radiology post-graduate secretary, for her friendliness, competence, good humor and willingness to help.

To Drs. **Carlos Malaguti, Moisés Vidal and Euda Pereira**, my colleagues who were exposed to radiation in the hemodynamics room at the **Francisca Mendes University Hospital in Manaus**. To the other colleagues and staff at this hospital, especially Dr. **Pedro Elias de Souza and Francisca Garcia**.

To my colleagues at **Santa Júlia Hospital**, especially Drs. **Edson Sarkis, Denise Nunes, Julia Gonçalves, Liane Cavalcante, Epifânio Pereira, Fabiana Lo Presti, Marcos Grangeiro, Luciano Santos, Denis Raid, Wander Ferreira, Rhea Motta and Vanise Amaral**.

To the secretaries **Télcia and Tania Loureiro**, for their attention and care for my patients.

To Dr. **Eurico Manoel Franco Azevedo**, who, while still an undergraduate at the **Federal University of Amazonas**, encouraged me to choose **Neurosurgery**; to the preceptors and fellow residents at the

Faculty of Medical Sciences of the Santa Casa de Sao Paulo, where I began my apprenticeship at Neurosurgery; to Dr.

Eduardo Ernesto Pelinca da Costa, who encouraged me to acquire a wonderful new subspecialty, **Interventional Neuroradiology**, and Professors **Serge Bracard, Rene Anxionnat, Luc Picard and Ariel Lebedinsky**, who taught me the neuroendovascular therapeutic method.

To the Faculty of Medicine of the University of Sao Paulo (FMUSP), for welcoming so well a researcher from another state, from another institution, who feels honored and will always honor the history of this House.

To **patients with AVMs**: understanding how to achieve their cure or clinical stabilization is the main objective of this work. Thank you for your confidence in the therapeutic method based on scientific evidence.

SUMMARY

Peres CMA. *Encephalic arteriovenous malformations: impact of nidal angioarchitecture on the outcome of radiosurgical treatment alone or preceded by embolization* .Sao Paulo: University of Sao Paulo School of Medicine; 2017.

Morphological aspects of the nerve and neoadjuvant partial embolization without the intention of curing encephalic arteriovenous malformations, preceding radiosurgery, may have an influence on the final outcome of the treatment. **Methods:** Consecutive series of 47 patients who underwent radiosurgery (1 to 5 sessions), preceded or not by cyanoacrylate embolization. Clinical and radiological follow-up of at least 36 months. **Results:** Hemorrhagic presentation occurred in 68.1% of the patients treated; of these, 62.5% had an arteriovenous fistula within the arteriovenous malformation; 83.3% venous ectasia and 90% restriction of venous drainage. The occlusion rate for embolization followed by radiosurgery was 46.1% and for radiosurgery alone was 52.4% (p=0.671). The following factors were identified as favoring occlusion: low nidal volume, absence of an intranidal arteriovenous fistula, higher radiation dose and low grade in the classification of brain arteriovenous malformations based on radiosurgery (RBAS). **Conclusions:** the smallest nidal volume (p<0.001), the lowest grade on the RBAS scale (p=0.047), the absence of an intranidal arteriovenous fistula (p=0.001) and the highest prescribed dose (p=0.001) were correlated with a favorable treatment outcome. Embolization followed by radiosurgery was not superior to radiosurgery alone (p=0.772). The elimination of intranidal arteriovenous fistulas by embolization may increase the effectiveness of radiosurgery.

Keywords: arteriovenous malformation of the brain; intracranial hemorrhage; endovascular procedures; therapeutic embolization; radiosurgery.

1 INTRODUCTION

Encephalic arteriovenous malformations (AVMs) are treated using four methods: expectant/symptomatic treatment, embolization, surgery and radiosurgery. The decision to treat invasively and the published studies on complications are based on the Spetzler-Martin classification[1,2], designed to stratify surgical risk. Thus, in the decision-making process, some important radiological and anatomical characteristics for the two other treatment methods (embolization and radiosurgery) are not taken into account, such as the occurrence of arteriovenous fistulas, venous ectasia, restriction of venous drainage due to stenosis or drainage by a single vein. The angioarchitecture of AVMs defined by these peculiar alterations in the vascular anatomy has so far not been correlated with the results of radiosurgery, preceded or not by embolization.

Partial embolization of the nidus is used to reduce the volume of extensive AVMs, as an adjuvant treatment to enable microsurgery or radiosurgery. However, the natural history of partially embolized AVMs, whether or not they are submitted to radiosurgery, is unknown and there are no defined protocols in the literature. In addition, there are no clear guidelines on how to proceed during embolization (it has not been defined what to embolize as a priority and what is not relevant to embolize).

2 OBJECTIVES

The primary objective of this study was:

To study the nidal, venous and arterial radiological changes associated with cerebral arteriovenous malformations, with the aim of correlating these changes with the outcome of combined treatment (endovascular followed by radiosurgery) or radiosurgery alone.

The secondary objectives were:

1.   To evaluate the effectiveness of radiosurgery associated or not with embolization in patients with cerebral arteriovenous malformations.

2.   To evaluate the effectiveness of prior embolization as an adjuvant therapy to radiosurgery treatment.

3.   To describe the population of patients with ruptured or non-ruptured AVMs who underwent treatment in the first 5 years of radiosurgery at the Radiology Institute of the Hospital das Clinicas of the University of Sao Paulo Medical School.

3 LITERATURE REVIEW

3.1 Definition

Encephalic arteriovenous malformations (AVMs) are cerebrovascular lesions characterized by the persistence of direct connections between arteries and veins, in the absence of a capillary bed, causing one or more arteriovenous fistulas in the same lesion[3,4]. The tangle of arterial and venous vessels that develops due to the high flow regime is called a **nido** (nest, in Latin), and represents the vascular lesion itself. High flow is the main hemodynamic alteration that promotes morphological changes and the eventual rupture of the malformation, resulting in intracranial hemorrhage. The term "encephalic arteriovenous malformation" has been used more frequently because it is more precise than "cerebral" (which excludes caudal structures) and "pial" (since many AVMs do not reach any pial surface)[4].

AVMs differ in topography, size, morphology and angioarchitecture. As such, treatment varies substantially from patient to patient. Despite the relatively low prevalence (15 cases per 100,000 inhabitants)[5] and incidence (1.12 cases per 100,000 inhabitants per year)[6] in the population, arteriovenous malformations are the main cause of non-traumatic intracranial hemorrhage in young patients (under 40 years of age)[7,8].

3.2 Natural history of the disease

AVMs can present clinically as:

-    Intracranial hemorrhage (with neurological deficit related to the intraparenchymal topography of the lesion or its extension into the subarachnoid or ventricular space) in 50% of cases.

-    Epileptic seizures in 30% of cases. They can be generalized or focal, in which case they may indicate the site of the lesion.

-    Headache in 14% of cases.

-    Other symptoms, such as focal neurological deficit (not related to bleeding, but due to the physical presence of the lesion or flow theft), pulsatile tinnitus or, occasionally, as an incidental finding in neuroimaging studies[9].

These percentages vary considerably depending on the geography of the populations studied: hemorrhage as a form of presentation in 71% of cases was found in the Nordic countries, and 42% and 52% in the United States and Europe, respectively[10].

The most common form of hemorrhage caused by a ruptured AVM is intraparenchymal, but in 24% of cases, subarachnoid and intraventricular hemorrhage can occur[11,12]. AVMs are usually single lesions, except when associated with hereditary hemorrhagic telangiectasia (Rendu-Osler-Weber disease)[13].

Ultimately, the decision on whether or not to treat an AVM must take into account the balance between the risks of intracranial hemorrhage and the risks of intervention. Unfortunately, the natural history of these malformations is still somewhat unknown, with numerous studies published, with marked heterogeneity, not only in the design of these studies, but also in the results[14]. The first studies were derived from surgical series and reported the percentage of patients with bleeding in a particular time interval[15]. More recent studies take into account an annual rate of bleeding and use multivariate analysis to differentiate between factors that can increase the risk independently and factors that are merely associated with the true predictive factor[16].

Intracranial hemorrhage was the most frequent form of presentation (65%) in the US state of Minessota in a population-based study by the Mayo Clinic. The incidence of the first hemorrhage was 0.82 per 100,000 person-years. The 30-day mortality rate for those who bled was 17.6%, with 75% of hemorrhages occurring under the age of 50[17].

Ondra[12] and colleagues, in a 24-year prospective study of 166 patients with symptomatic AVMs (not all of whom presented with bleeding), found an annual bleeding rate of 4% per year and a mortality rate of 1% per year. At the end of the study, 23% of the patients had died from bleeding.

The Ondra study was, for decades (and is still widely cited and used), the cornerstone of the natural history of AVMs. However, in addition to the limitation mentioned above (of mixing ruptured AVMs with non-ruptured AVMs), the study ended in 1975, and computed tomography became commercially available in 1973; therefore, many of the "hemorrhagic" cases were detected only by symptomatology or by lumbar puncture[18].

Taking into account an annual bleeding risk of between 2 and 4% in non-routed AVMs, the risk of bleeding could be calculated using the formula[9,19,20]:

Risk of bleeding (%) = 105 - age.

This formula was drawn up assuming a homogeneous population and does not take into account the appearance of risk factors such as aneurysms associated with AVMs.

Hernesniemi and colleagues studied 238 consecutive patients with untreated AVM, from admission (the first in 1942) to the start of treatment or hemorrhage or death or until the end of recruitment in 2005. Clinical follow-up ranged from 1 month to 53 years (average 13.5 years). The annual rate of bleeding was 2.4%. The risk factors identified were: early age, previous rupture, deep, infratentorial locations and exclusive deep venous drainage[21].

The Columbia AVM Database project and the New York Islands AVM Study[22,23], in a prospective analysis of 600 patients, found:

- annual bleeding rate of 34.4% in patients with 3 risk factors at the same time: previous bleeding, deep location and deep venous drainage;

- in patients with previous bleeding, but without either of these two risk factors, the rate was 4.5%;

- in those who had never bled, the annual bleeding rate was 3.1% for deep AVMs, 2.4% for AVMs with deep venous drainage and 0.9% for patients with non-routed AVMs without either of these two risk factors[18].

The prospective, multicenter "Randomized Study of Non-Routable AVMs" ("*ARUBA*") showed that clinical treatment was superior to intervention (surgery, radiosurgery or embolization). The study recruited only 226 of the 400 planned patients, as it was stopped early by the "*safety board*" - an independent monitoring committee appointed by the *NIH* (US National Institute of Health), since the primary outcome, defined as symptomatic cerebrovascular accident or death, was observed in 10% of the cohort submitted to clinical treatment and 31% in the group submitted to intervention (p<0.0001), over an average follow-up of 33 months[24].

This study has raised numerous discussions about its external validity (difficulty in generalizing the results of this study to other populations), especially due to the heterogeneous mix of lesions (including high-risk AVMs and low-risk AVMs) and the interventions carried out. Despite being randomized, the study suffered from a strong selection bias, especially when it came to recruitment, since many centers in the United States, even though they agreed to take part in the study, claimed that there was no clinical justification for judging that there was not enough doubt *not to treat, but to randomize* a significant number of patients who had high risk factors for a non-routine AVM[25].

In a meta-analysis recently published by Harvard Medical School[14], including 3,923 patients and 18,423 patient-years of follow-up, the annual rate of bleeding in non-ruptured AVMs was 2.2% (95% CI between 1.7% and 2.7%) and, for ruptured AVMs, it was 4.5% (95% CI between 3.7% and 5.5%). These figures are highly influenced by the risk factors that will be described below, and may have minimal significance for a particular AVM[14].

3.3 Pathophysiology

AVMs can be part of a neurological syndrome in 2% of cases. This group includes hereditary hemorrhagic telangiectasia (Osler-Weber-Rendu disease) and cerebrofacial arteriovenous metameric syndromes[26]. In the case of sporadic AVMs, which are the most common, the traditional etiopathogenic hypothesis is based on observations of the normal development of cerebral circulation.

They originate during the period of intrauterine development when the embryo is 4 to 8 cm long (approximately 10 to 14 weeks of gestation), when the processes of vasculogenesis and angiogenesis are in full swing[27].

However, various pieces of evidence have challenged this traditional concept, suggesting that AVMs, like dural arteriovenous fistulas, are acquired lesions:

- the average age of clinical detection follows a normal distribution curve, with a peak at the age of 40[7].

- Routine prenatal ultrasound scans, which detect lesions already present at birth (such as aneurysmal malformation of the vein of Galen and dural sinus malformations with arteriovenous fistula), do not detect encephalic AVMs[28].

- in the last two decades, with the advent of high-resolution resonance imaging, numerous reports have been described of *de novo* AVMs (in patients who did not have this lesion on previous images)[29,30].

- AVMs can develop in experimental models (adult mice) under certain conditions[31].

This evidence suggests that AVMs are not static congenital defects, but undergo active vascular alterations (angiogenesis and vascular remodeling) with the potential for postnatal onset or growth. The exact mechanism would include:

- abnormalities in the groups of regulatory genes ("*homeobox*") involved in angiogenesis[32];

- abnormalities in cell signaling (necessary for the regulation of cell organization, such as *Notch-4* transmembrane proteins, which are receptors that promote the expression of arterial molecular markers and suppress venous markers; *Notch* activity in the endothelium would be aberrantly increased in AVMs[33];

- a factor, or environmental trigger, that would lead to a disorganization in vascular proliferation[34]. Venous hypertension (which could occur in a localized area of microvascular thrombosis such as a minor head trauma) could induce the formation of AVMs through various mechanisms, as in the pathophysiology of dural arteriovenous fistulas[35].

The pathogenesis of AVM rupture is also not clearly understood, but there are studies that point to inflammation as one of the main factors[36]. Single nucleotide genetic polymorphisms would cause a positive modulation ("*up-regulation*") of inflammatory cytokines, which would induce an increase in the expression of adhesion molecules in endothelial cells, resulting in the recruitment of leukocytes. These, in turn, would release matrix metalloproteinase-9 (MMP-9), an extracellular matrix enzyme that degrades type IV collagen and is implicated in vascular remodeling under normal and pathological circumstances. An increase in this enzyme would damage the vascular wall of the AVM, causing rupture[37].

Inhibition of the vascular degradation activity of MMP-9 is one of the potential therapeutic targets for preventing bleeding in AVMs. Hashimoto et al. studied 14 patients with AVMs, 10 of whom received doxycycline (an antibiotic that reduces MMP-9 levels) and 4 of whom received placebo. After surgical removal of AVMs, a reduction in MMP-9 levels was observed in the resected specimens of patients who received doxycycline[38,39].

Chronic high flow produces secondary structural alterations in the nourishing arteries and draining veins, and is associated with the formation of arterial aneurysms and venous ectasias. Aneurysms are present in 2.3% to 16.7% of AVMs[40]. These aneurysms can be proximal (arteries of the Willis polygon), distal or nidal[41]. Proximal aneurysms are easier to detect on routine diagnostic angiography and have a higher incidence in the elderly and in the posterior circulation[42].

The detection of nidal aneurysms often depends on selective microcatheterization, and the incidence can be even higher than described above when this technique is used[43]. For some authors, nidal aneurysms are venous aneurysms, as the nidus consists of a tangle of structures that are histopathologically more related to veins[43,44]. For other authors, nidal aneurysms would be false aneurysms originating from the dysplastic vessels that form the nidus, and would represent the exact bleeding site of an AVM[45,46].

Arteriovenous fistulas, consisting of direct connections between arteries and veins (without nidal interposition) may be present within the AVM. Microfistulas are generally only identified on superselective angiography (performed with microcatheters). The angioarchitecture of the nidus can be formed by a plexiform network, direct fistulas between the nourishing artery and the draining vein or a mixed plexiform pattern with fistulas[47].

Venous ectasias are seen in AVMs with reduced drainage and are considered a risk factor for hemorrhage. Hemorrhage would occur due to rupture of the nidal vessels, most commonly the draining vein due to increased pressure or thrombosis. It could also occur due to rupture of associated aneurysms[48].

High flow in large AVMs could generate a phenomenon of arterial "flow theft" in neighboring healthy brain tissue, leading to neurological deficits (motor, visual, cognitive) without evidence of bleeding[49]. However, this concept has not been proven in intra-arterial pressure and flow measurements[50].

3.4   Risk factors for bleeding

AVMs are heterogeneous lesions, with a large number of factors that can influence the risk of hemorrhage. In order to identify these factors, studies using multivariate analysis are important to differentiate between those that independently predict risk and others that are merely associated with the true predictive factor[10]. For example, it was believed that AVMs with a small nidus had a higher risk of bleeding[51], however, a Finnish prospective study showed that a larger nidus is a predictive factor of future bleeding[52]. Similarly, since bleeding as a form of presentation is more frequent in children, it was believed that early age was a risk factor for subsequent bleeding. In an extensive study, it was shown that the risk of future bleeding was lower in children than in adults[53].

Statistically significant risk factors for bleeding in an AVM include[14,54]:

- Bleeding as the initial presentation: annual rate of rebleeding between 9.65% and 15.42%[10,18,23].

- Deep AVMs (thalamus and basal ganglia) and brainstem AVMs. Although they account for 10% and 5% of AVMs, respectively, these lesions have a more aggressive natural history, manifesting as bleeding at the time of diagnosis in 72% to 91% of cases[23,55].

- Exclusive deep venous drainage, although more studies are needed, as there is a coincidence between this characteristic and the deep location and hemorrhagic presentation of AVMs. The annual risk of bleeding when deep venous drainage and deeply located AVM coincide is 8%, and deep venous drainage and hemorrhage as the initial presentation is 11.4% per year[10,52].

- Associated aneurysms occur in 2.3% to 16.7% of AVMs[40] and are considered risk factors for hemorrhage with an *odds ratio of* 1.8 (95% confidence interval 1.6-2.0)[14]. This risk would be higher in aneurysms of distal or intranidal feeding vessels. Proximal aneurysms do not seem to be related to AVM hemorrhage[56].

3.5 Diagnosis

Non-contrast-enhanced computed tomography (CT) effectively diagnoses bleeding, but has low sensitivity (50% to 77%) for detecting AVM itself, and can show calcifications and hypodense areas. With the use of iodinated contrast, AVMs can be detected through a serpiginous pattern of contrast enhancement. CT angiography (Figure 1) can provide three-dimensional information in selected cases[9,57].

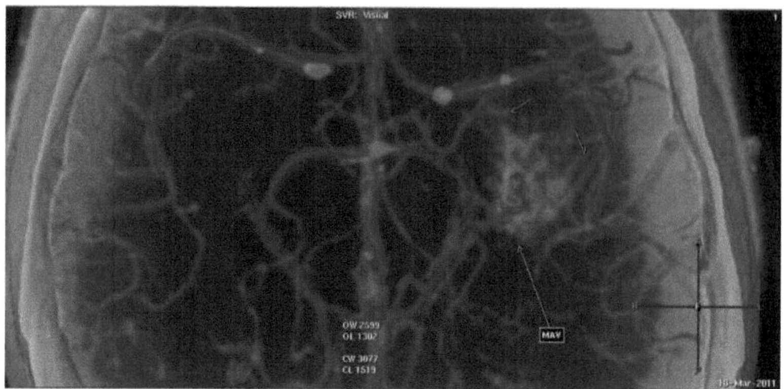

Figure 1 - Angiotomography of AVM in the left basal ganglia.

Magnetic resonance imaging (MRI) is more sensitive, showing "*flow* voids" and hemosiderin deposits on T1- and T2-weighted images. Only in cases of small calcified malformations is CT superior to MRI. The specificity of MRI can be affected by the similarity between some highly vascularized neoplasms (such as some glioblastomas) and AVMs, especially if there is hemorrhage from the latter with perilesional edema[57]. MRI evaluation is essential to determine the precise topography and the relationship of the lesion with eloquent areas of the brain parenchyma[58].

Magnetic resonance angiography can provide information such as the nature of the nourishing arteries and draining veins. However, it has limitations when it comes to assessing the flow *and* details of venous and arterial anatomy, and the presence of associated lesions such as intranidal aneurysms[59].

Digital cerebral angiography is the most accurate method for delineating AVM angioarchitecture, providing information on hemodynamics, including flow velocity, node size, arterial supply and venous drainage. Superselective injection of AVM afferents using microcatheters reveals more information, such as the presence of aneurysms and direct arteriovenous fistulas within the nerve[60].

Pollock *et al.*[61], evaluating the accuracy of resonance imaging compared to angiography after radiosurgery for AVMs, compared the visualization of *flow voids* on pre-radiosurgery MRI in 164 patients with post-radiosurgery, concluding that MRI is a suitable non-invasive method for evaluating the response to treatment. Evidence of AVM occlusion on MRI images was defined as the absence of *flow-void* on proton density, T1 and T2 weightings. Thus, resonance imaging is used to more adequately determine the optimal time to obtain digital angiography images, which is considered the gold standard for determining vascular exclusion (radioanatomical cure) of the lesion[62].

For treatment planning purposes, it is necessary to calculate the volume of AVMs with a reasonable margin of accuracy. Different formulas are used to calculate the volume of the malformation, all based on the triplanar linear dimension. Brown[63] calculates AVM volume as an elongated sphere:

Volume = 4/3 π (1/2 S)^3+ ¼ π. S^{2}X (L-S)

In this formula, S is the smallest and L is the largest diameter of the sphere.

The "ellipsoid method" was developed to calculate the volume based on the concept that the ellipsoid is approximately half the volume of the parallelepiped (a polyhedron with six faces, which are parallelograms in pairs of parallel planes). By measuring three diameters of a given lesion in the arterial phase of angiography, the parallelepiped is constructed and its volume, divided by two, is close to the real volume of the malformation[59].

Considering A, B and C as the 3 diameters of the AVM (width, height and depth), the ellipsoid formula is:

Volume of the ellipsoid = 4/3π. [(A/2).(B/2).(C/2)]

If we assume that π =3, the formula becomes:

AVM volume = (A . B. C) /2

For practical purposes, the volume can be calculated, without too much loss of accuracy, using the latter formula[64-66]. Thus, a 2cm diameter AVM would have an approximate volume of 4cm^3 and a 4.6cm AVM would have an approximate volume of 50cm^3.

The angiographic criteria for defining the angioarchitecture of AVMs were systematized in *"Reporting Terminology for Brain Arteriovenous Malformations Clinical and Radiological Features for Use in Clinical Trials"*, in which a task force tried to standardize terminology that was previously quite confusing and heterogeneous[4].

3.6   Treatment: decision and evaluation of response

Considering the neurological devastation caused by intracranial hemorrhage caused by the rupture of an AVM, the primary goal of treatment is the complete removal or obliteration of the nerve[67], while preserving the function and structure of the adjacent brain tissue. Successful treatment of these malformations remains a challenge, even with the isolated or combined use of available therapies: microsurgical resection, embolization and radiosurgery[68,69].

The angiographic criteria used for response to treatment include 4 subgroups[4,70]:

1. Healing: no evidence of a nidus or draining vein.

2. Subtotal occlusion: no evidence of nido, but with a visible draining vein, suggesting the existence of an arteriovenous *shunt*.

3.   Partial occlusion: obliteration of 50 to 90% of the nerve.

4.   Minimum response: reduction of the fluid by 10 to 50% of the initial volume.

The results of partial treatment of an AVM are controversial in the literature, but most authors consider that it does not prevent bleeding and can have worse effects than the natural history of the disease[71,72]. Raupp *et al.* showed, in a multivariate analysis, that embolization of less than 2/3 would not protect the patient from rebleeding from the AVM[72].

There is a risk of recurrence even after angiographic follow-up has demonstrated total eradication of the AVM[73]. Younger patients (under 18) and the presence of deep venous drainage seem to be the main factors[74] associated with recurrence. In the pediatric population, it is postulated that immature vessels can enter into active angiogenesis; high local levels of VEGF have been demonstrated in patients with AVM recurrence[75].

Treatment by microsurgical resection is the most effective way of immediately eliminating the risk of hemorrhage[76,77]. It offers immediate elimination of the risk of hemorrhage, treats the symptoms of vascular steal and often improves the control of seizures. However, certain large AVMs in eloquent or deep regions of the brain are not amenable to microsurgery due to the unacceptable morbidity and mortality rate associated with this type of treatment. For such lesions, the alternatives are embolization and/or radiosurgery[78].

3.6.1 Scales

Deciding on the most appropriate course of action for an arteriovenous malformation is often complex, as it includes factors such as previous bleeding (or not), the characteristics of the AVM and the patient. As the natural history of this disease is still somewhat unknown, the identification of predictive factors and the development of scales allow for a risk-benefit analysis and the comparison of results between possible forms of treatment. According to Spetzler and Martin, the sum of the points of the criteria presented in Table 1 will stratify AVMs into grades from 1 to 5. This grade would be proportional to the difficulty in surgically treating AVMs[1].

Chart 1 - Spetzler-Martin (SM) classification of encephalic arteriovenous malformations (1986).

Criteria	Features	Points
Size	< 3cm	1
	3 - 6cm	2
	> 6cm	3
Eloquence of the adjacent brain area	Not eloquent	0
	Eloquent	1
Venous drainage	Only superficial	0

	Deep	1

On this scale, deep veins are those that drain into the internal cerebral veins, the basal vein of Rosenthal and the pre-central cerebellar vein. In the posterior fossa, only the hemispheric cerebellar veins that drain directly into the straight sinus, torcula or transverse sinus are considered superficial drainage (all the others are considered deep)[4].

The following brain areas are considered eloquent: primary sensory-motor cortex, language cortex and visual cortex; hypothalamus, thalamus, internal capsule, brainstem, cerebellar peduncles and deep cerebellar nuclei.

The classification was revised in 1988 by Oliveira[2], who subdivided grade III into:

- IIIA: grade 3 AVM due to size, greater than 3cm;

- IIIB: grade 3 AVM due to its location in an eloquent area, with a diameter of less than 3cm.

It is generally accepted that patients with grade I and II AVMs should be treated with surgery, and grade IV and V with a multidisciplinary approach. Grade IIIA AVMs should be treated with embolization to reduce their size and then treated by surgery or radiosurgery. Grade IIIB AVMs should be treated with radiosurgery[70].

The modification introduced by Spetzler and Ponce[79] did not bring any major practical changes, combining grades I and II (Class A), grade III (Class B), and grades IV and V (Class C).

As the Spetzler-Martin scale was developed to predict the outcome of AVM treatment by conventional surgery, it was observed that not all the elements of the scale are predictive of the final outcome[80] and that there was no correlation with radiosurgery treatment, as it did not include factors such as specific sites and the patient's age[70,81,82].

In an attempt to predict the outcome of radiosurgery for arteriovenous malformations, Pollock and Flickinger, at the University of Pittsburgh, developed a score in 2002[83] (modified[84] in 2008), using multivariate analysis of factors involved in the outcome of the treatment of irradiated AVMs . This scale, known as the *"radiosurgery-based AVM score"* (RBAS), includes the patient's age (in years), the volume of the AVM (in cubic centimeters) and the topography of the lesion. Some studies have shown that this scale has good accuracy in predicting the outcome of radiosurgery in AVMs [85-87]. Other studies have shown that there was no difference between this scale and the Spetzler-Martin scale[88,89].

Using demographic data and data on the volume and location of the AVM according to the MRI scan, the lesions are classified using the RBAS scale as shown in Table 2:

Table 2 - Classification of brain arteriovenous malformations based on radiosurgery, according to

Pollock and Flickinger

Criteria	Factor (multiply by)
AVM volume (ml)	0,1
Patient's age (years)	0,02
Surface topography	0
Deep topography (basal nuclei, thalamus or brainstem)	1

According to these criteria, the degree of AVM is calculated according to the equation:

RBAS grade = 0.1. (volume) + 0.02. (age) + 0.5. (topography)

According to the results of this scale, the chances of a satisfactory outcome (occlusion of the AVM without new deficits) would be[84]:

Grade < 1: 89%; between 1.01 and 1.50: 70%; between 1.51 and 2: 64%; greater than 2: 46%

3.6.2 Embolization

Embolization aims to achieve vascular occlusion of the AVM, preserving the arterial supply and venous drainage of the surrounding normal brain parenchyma. Depending on the angioarchitecture and location of the lesion, the endovascular therapeutic procedure includes transarterial or superselective transvenous microcatheterization. After positioning the microcatheter in a preferably intranidal situation, the primary objective is to occlude the nerve or part of it and, ideally, the beginning of the drainage vena and the nourishing arteriole[90]. This occlusion is achieved with the use of embolizing agents[91,92].

The search for the ideal embolizing agent is a challenge that persists in therapeutic neuroradiology[91,93]. The first report of embolization of an arteriovenous malformation dates back to 1960, when Luessenhop and Spence described the use of methylmethacrylate embolic spheres[94]; since then, a variety of particles have been used[95], which, although effective in some cases, had a low degree of occlusion and/or a high degree of repermeabilization, undesirable venous passage or proximal occlusion[96].

The advent of embolizing liquids was what brought about the greatest advance in the endovascular treatment of AVMs, because while before catheters at least as wide as microparticles were needed, with liquids (developed to solidify once inside the AVM's node), it became possible to use much thinner microcatheters[91].

Cyanoacrylate embolization, when correctly indicated and carried out, can be curative, with the degree of permanent occlusion of the embolized vessels being the same as that of the AVM. If the initial angiography after treatment indicates a cure, this usually translates into a permanent cure.

However, in the series published in the most current literature, only 10 to 51% of patients are curable by the endovascular method alone. Angiographic characteristics such as multiple arterial supplies and/or "*en passant*" vessels, which also irrigate normal brain tissue, are one of the main limitations of the method[97].

There is evidence[98] that partial occlusion of an AVM by endovascular means could lead to an undesirable increase in angiogenesis, through 3 mechanisms:

1)   Local hypoxia caused by the occlusion of small vessels and the consequent endothelial release of vascular growth factor (VEGF) and hypoxia-induced factor (HIF-1), which spread, causing the *sprouting* of new vessels.

2)   Acute and chronic inflammatory reaction caused by embolizing agents, with the release of interleukin-6 (the main inflammatory cytokine, which is also angiogenic).

3)   Increased flow with vascular stress in neighboring vessels that have not been obliterated, which also releases VEGF and induces the expression of fetal liver kinase-1 (which is a VEGF receptor) in the endothelium[98].

Prior embolization of an AVM could reduce cure rates in radiosurgery[99-101]. However, there are no prospective or randomized studies to prove this and, in most published studies, there are limitations such as a strong selection bias when indicating embolization followed by radiosurgery for patients with larger AVMs and more complex angioarchitecture[102]. The percentage of Spetzler-Martin grades III to V was higher in the embolized group than in the non-embolized group in the Andrade-Souza study[99]. The volume of AVMs in the embolized group was significantly greater than in the non-embolized group in the studies by Xu[100] and Back[101].

The use of tantalum, a high atomic number material (Z=73) used to provide radiopacity, would cause a "shielding" effect in some compartments of the AVM. In a study with an experimental model[103], this effect did not cause a significant reduction in the dose delivered to the center of the model, as it would be compensated for by the dispersive effect and the multiple entry points inherent in the radiotherapy treatment itself.

In addition to these factors, the beneficial effects of embolization in reducing the incidence of radiation-induced complications and reducing the risk of hemorrhage in the latency period after radiosurgery for occlusion to occur have not been studied[100].

In cases of embolization as a neoadjuvant treatment (pre-radiosurgery or pre-surgery), complications seem to be related to the attempt at nidal embolization[104]. Associated or causal factors of such complications include microperforations, hemodynamic changes after embolization, significant venous occlusion, rupture of intranidal aneurysms and persistent intranidal venous stagnation[105].

Embolization can only be used to treat fragile points in the AVM, such as arteriovenous fistulas, as long as it is done using a technique that allows the junction between the feeding artery and the beginning of the venous component (the site of the fistula) to be located. As it is often necessary to occlude this venous component, it is necessary to ensure that the kidney has other drainage routes. Other times, it is necessary to use micromoles to reduce the flow, preventing the embolizing liquid from migrating to the distal venous system, such as cerebral veins, dural sinuses or even pulmonary circulation. Radiosurgical obliteration of non-nidal (non-"plexiform") components of an arteriovenous malformation is statistically lower than that of the nidus, reinforcing the indication for embolization in these cases [81,104].

Embolization of large AVMs (those larger than $10cm^3$), with the aim of reducing the size of the node to a volume suitable for radiosurgery, should target the compartments at the periphery of the AVM [78,102], reducing the volume to a compact node. The endovascular strategy used to reduce flow, which is advocated in preoperative embolization, should be avoided, as diffuse embolization of the node makes radiotherapy planning difficult by dissociating the target into several irregular clusters [82,99,106,107].

3.6.3 Radiosurgery

Radiosurgery aims to damage precisely defined areas of the brain with radiation, usually in a single session, but which can be divided into up to 5 sessions. In practical terms, the vast majority of current radiosurgery procedures are carried out using photon sources: with a *"Gamma Knife"* or a linear particle accelerator (LINAC)[108].

"Stereotactic radiosurgery" was conceptually introduced by Swedish neurosurgeon Lars Leksell in 1951, initially to treat movement disorders and chronic pain with high doses of energy from photons, culminating in the creation, in 1967, of stereotactic equipment for administering multiple foci of cobalt 60 sources, the *"Gamma Knife"* (GK). In the first decades of its use, stereotactic localization depended on the use of topographic atlases, pneumoencephalograms or cerebral angiographies. Leksell himself was one of the pioneers in the use of spatial information from tomography and MRI, which gave a new and definitive impetus to the stereotactic method. Over the last six decades, this method has established itself as a suitable treatment for AVMs, or even as the only option in some cases. It offers a minimally invasive alternative to surgical resection, especially in deep lesions or those located in neurologically significant areas[109,110].

Using the same principles as GK, in the 1980s, Betti *et al.*[111] pioneered the use of linear accelerator radiosurgery (LINAC)[112], using microwave energy to accelerate electrons and make them collide with a heavy metal alloy. Part of this energy is converted into photons (identical to those used in GK). By rotating the device at different angles, a series of converging arcs is obtained, with dose distribution and clinical results similar to those obtained by GK[113].

The histopathological changes caused by radiosurgery initially include endothelial damage, which induces the proliferation of smooth muscle cells in the intima. These produce extracellular matrix (type IV collagen), causing hyperplasia of the intima, progressive luminal narrowing and obliteration of the AVM node. This cellular degeneration and hyaline transformation are similar to the atherosclerosis model[114]. Fibrosis in the adventitia composed of type IV collagen and smooth muscle cells in between has also been detected in models of porcine *"rete mirabile"* submitted to radiosurgery[115].

The aim of radiosurgery is to obliterate the AVM node, eliminating the risk of future bleeding. Complete obliteration of the nidus usually takes between 1 and 3 years[116-119]. The risk of bleeding during this long latency period remains unchanged compared to untreated patients[119-121]. In another study, radiosurgery significantly reduced the risk of bleeding in patients with AVMs, even before there was evidence of angiographic obliteration[122]. In addition, conditions such as radiation-induced necrosis, edema and cerebral cysts can occur later[88].

The rate of AVM obliteration after radiosurgery varies in the literature[116-118,123-125] from 50 to 92%. In studies using multivariate analysis, the diameter/volume of the nidus, the number of drainage veins, the marginal dose, the Spetzler-Martin grade, the presence of dilated afferent vessels and the flow (presence of a fast fistula) had some influence on the final result[123,125].

Radiation-induced complications after radiosurgery can occur transiently in 5-11% of patients and result in permanent neurological deficits in 1-3% of cases[82].

Confirmation by MRI and angiography that an AVM is obliterated by radiosurgery may not mean a definitive absence of hemorrhagic risk[126], especially in children[127] The possible mechanism to explain this is the early thickening of the endothelium in small-caliber nidal vessels. When blood flow falls below the level detectable by angiography, the AVM becomes invisible, although it is still histologically present[122].

Classically, radiosurgery has been applied[128] to lesions up to 3cm in diameter or smaller than 10cm^3. The risk-benefit ratio of radiosurgery for large AVMs has traditionally been reported as unfavorable, with low rates of obliteration and high rates of radiation-induced complications[129]. Considering that the degree of obliteration is directly linked to the total dose of radiation used, treating large AVMs with traditionally effective doses of radiation can result in a risk of adverse radiological effects on adjacent brain tissue[130].

Due to these limitations, some AVMs require radiosurgery in five fractions and/or prior embolization[131,132]. Various strategies have been described, generally with fractionated radiosurgery at intervals of 6 to 9 months and 3 to 4 years for repeat radiosurgery, in an effort to reduce the deleterious effects of radiation and promote AVM obliteration[133].

Embolization followed by radiosurgery is another approach. The aim is to perform one or more sessions of non-curative embolization to reduce the size of the AVM, followed by radiosurgery to treat the remaining tissue, allowing the treatment of AVMs that were initially too bulky for isolated radiosurgical treatment[66,134,135].

The delineation of the nidus in patients with previously embolized AVMs can be difficult. One possible reason is that portions of the nidus remain scattered among the original volume, masked by the Onyx ball (which causes a strong radiological artifact due to the presence of tantalum in its composition) or cyanoacrylate[106,134] New liquid embolizing agents, such as PHIL (*Precipitating Hydrophobic* Injectable Liquid), are being introduced, which are less radiopaque but still provide good radioscopic visualization, with the aim of reducing artifacts in neuroimaging exams[91,136].

4 METHODS

4.1 Study design

The study and its informed consent form were approved by the Department of Radiology and Oncology of the HCFMUSP, and by the Ethics Committee for the Analysis of Research Projects (CAPPesq) of the HCFMUSP, report number 522.359 (Annexes A, B and C).

This was a single-center, longitudinal cohort study based on retrospective observation of clinical records and digital image files from the Radiology Institute (InRad) of the Hospital das Clinicas of the Faculty of Medicine of the University of São Paulo (HCFMUSP) and the application of a prospective protocol over the last three years (Appendix D). The recruitment period was from July 2008 to December 2012, allowing angiographic controls (when indicated) until December 2015.

4.2 Casuistry

Patients were admitted and assessed at a joint meeting of the Neurosurgery, Therapeutic Neuroradiology and Radiotherapy Departments at HCFMUSP. The criteria for not indicating surgical removal and indicating radiosurgery and/or embolization were assessed on a case-by-case basis, respecting the patient's wishes.

All the patients included in this study underwent a clinical assessment in the Radiosurgery Department, with clinical data recorded in electronic or manual medical records which were then digitized.

The medical records containing clinical data, treatments and outpatient follow-ups, as well as the images stored in the PACS (*Picture Archiving and Communication System*) system, were sequentially reviewed, preserving the confidentiality of the sources of information.

Demographic data, clinical history, changes in the neurological and neuroimaging examination, the nature and results of the treatments the patients underwent were taken into account.

4.2.1 Inclusion criteria

1.   Patients diagnosed with brain arteriovenous malformation (AVM), under International Classification of Diseases (ICD) Q 28.2, with the data from the protocol (Appendix D).

2.   Patients who have undergone stereotactic radiosurgery preceded or not by embolization, with a minimum follow-up of 3 years, or who have been investigated with MRI with a suggestion of occlusion before the 3th year and with angiography showing complete obliteration of the AVM.

4.2.2 Exclusion criteria

1.   Patients undergoing neurosurgical treatment for AVM.

2.   Patients without neuroimaging exams or of poor technical quality, preventing analysis of the hemodynamics and angioarchitecture of the AVM (for example, making it impossible to measure venous drainage).

3.   Patients without clinical and radiological follow-up in the first 3 years after radiosurgery.

4.2.3 Variables

4.2.3.1 Independent variables

a)   Clinical and demographic data:

Data was systematically collected from the medical records of eligible patients: identification, age, gender, initial and final neurological examination, from which the modified Rankim scale was derived (Appendix E). The duration, in months, of the last angiographic (when indicated) and magnetic resonance imaging (in all) controls was recorded.

b)   Arteriovenous Malformation Data:

According to the MRI, CT and angiography images, the volume and topography of the AVM were recorded and classified as eloquent or non-eloquent separately.

Spetzler-Martin scores[2] and the modified Pollock-Flickinger scale[84] (RBAS, *Radiosurgery-Based AVM Scale*) were calculated.

Arterial characteristics (number of nourishing arteries, presence and type of aneurysms) and venous characteristics (restrictive alteration to the venous blood flow of the arteriovenous malformation, according to angiographic parameters: reduced number of draining veins, venous stenosis, venous dilation and deep venous drainage exclusively) were also noted.

4.2.3.2 Dependent variables

The primary dependent variable was considered to be the outcome of the treatment according to the angiographic cure of the AVM.

The secondary dependent variables were: the occurrence of bleeding complications (the presence of recent bleeding was assessed with T2* weighting).

(T2 "star")) or ischemic after radiosurgery treatment and the change in the neurological examination according to the modified Rankin scale (Appendix E).

4.3 Definitions

1.   Definition of an arteriovenous fistula within an AVM[104]:

-      Dilated nourishing artery (diameter greater than twice that of arteries supplying corresponding contralateral areas) directly connected to a venous component.

- Absence of plexiform nidus/component between artery and vein.

- Dural arteriovenous fistulas or "pial" arteriovenous fistulas unrelated to AVMs are not part of this definition.

2. Definition of a feeding artery:

Structure that angiographically demonstrates a contribution to AVM flow, according to contrast opacification[4].

3. Definition of AVM-related arterial aneurysm:

Saccular dilatations of arteries supplying the AVM, usually caused by flow[4]. They can be *intranidal* (when inside or adjacent to the nerve), *proximal* or *distal*. The latter two terms refer to the Willis polygon: "proximal" includes the internal carotid arteries, basilar arteries and the trunks of the anterior, middle or posterior cerebral arteries.

4. Definition of venous stenosis:

Narrowing of the draining vein in two angiographic planes, with a reduction in diameter of more than 50% when compared to the same vessel after AVM exit[125,137].

5. Definition of venous ectasia:

A greater than twofold increase in diameter in a draining vein[4] (Figure 2). If there is no uniformity in venous caliber, the diameter of the vein at its exit from the nidus should be used as a reference.

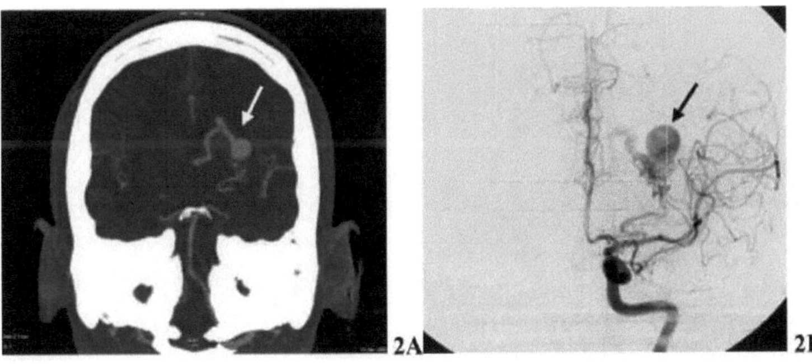

Figure 2 - Venous ectasia seen on angiotomography (arrow) (A) and digital cerebral angiography (arrow) (B).

6. Definition of suggested cure by MRI: absence of *flow-void* in proton density, Tl and T2 weightings[61].

7. Definition of angiographic cure and other outcomes[4,70]:

- **Cure**: complete absence of abnormal vessels forming in the tissue, normal circulatory time and absence of arteriovenous fistula. Figure 3 shows a parieto-occipital AVM, with previous hemorrhage, treated with radiosurgery in 2012, with angiographic control in 2015 showing cure.

- **Subtotal occlusion**: no evidence of a nidus, but with a visible draining vein, suggesting the existence of an arteriovenous fistula.

- **Partial occlusion**: obliteration of 50 to 90% of the nerve.

- **Minimum response**: reduction of the fluid by 10 to 50% of the initial volume.

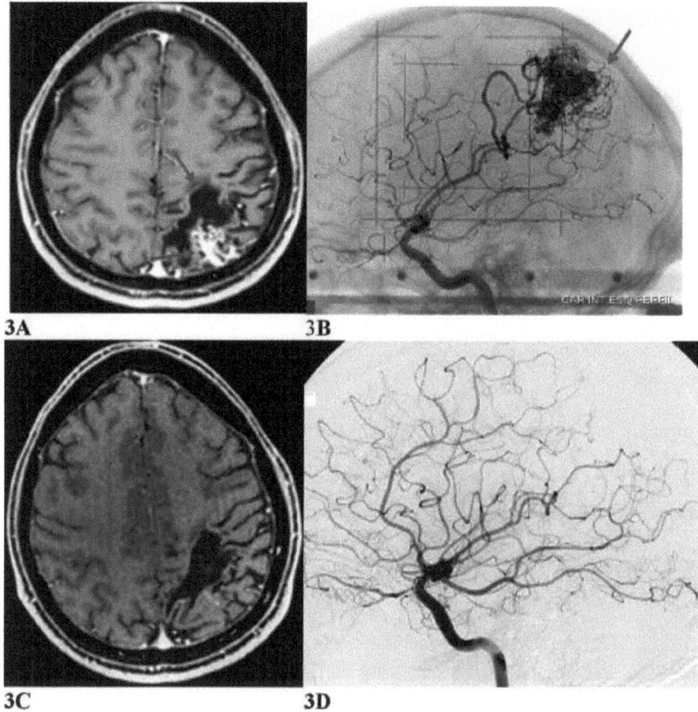

Figure 3 - Parieto-occipital AVM with a history of hemorrhage (encephalomalacia - blue arrow in A, and nido - red arrow in A and B). She underwent radiosurgery in 2012. MRI (C) and 2015 control angiography (D) show no lesion.

8. Definition of radiation-induced radiological alteration:

Transient or definitive, symptomatic or asymptomatic hypersignal on T2 and FLAIR. Symptomatic and definitive lesions with paramagnetic contrast impregnation characterize radionecrosis[88].

9. Definition of favorable outcome of radiosurgery treatment:

Complete angiographic occlusion of the AVM, no symptomatic radiation-induced changes and no post-treatment bleeding[138].

4.4 Embolization

The embolizations were performed under general anesthesia in the Interventional Radiology Department of the Radiology Institute of the University of Sao Paulo Medical School. A senior neuroradiologist was always in charge of the procedures, which aimed to reduce the volume of the AVM, typically to a diameter of less than 3cm. Embolization also aimed to eliminate or reduce more fragile abnormalities in the AVM, such as direct arteriovenous fistulas and arterial and venous aneurysms.

The *Seldinger* technique[139] was used to catheterize the right femoral artery. A 6F or 5F diameter introducer was used to pass 6F or 5F catheters which, aided by 0.035 inch hydrophilic guides, were positioned in the vessels of the cervical region (carotid or vertebral). Confirmatory angiographic series were carried out, allowing the best incidence to be studied and the pedicles most suitable for embolization to be selected.

Next, 1.5F caliber microcatheters aided by microguides were navigated coaxially, performing superselective catheterization of the afferent arterioles of the AVM. When properly positioned in abnormal arteries (confirmed by angiographic microseries), the microcatheters were perfused with 5% glucose saline (to avoid polymerization inside them) and then injected with Lipiodol and n-butyl-cyanoacrylate (NBCA) solution, in proportions that varied according to flow and the presence or absence of a rapid arteriovenous fistula. Lipiodol, a fatty contrast based on poppy oil, also serves to dilute the NBCA, increasing or decreasing the speed of polymerization, depending on the speed of flow in the AVM.

4.5 Radiosurgery

All the patients underwent 1.5T MRI using Gadolinium paramagnetic contrast in a volume of 10ml. The MRI was carried out in the same week, prior to the day of the radiosurgery.

In patients treated with a single dose, the stereotactic equipment fixed to the cephalic segment was used, making it possible to locate the targets (AVMs) for the radiosurgery. This procedure was performed under local anesthesia in adults and under general anesthesia in children.

For those treated with 5 fractions, a stereotactic mask (made of thermo-moldable material and adjusted individually for each patient) was made about a week before the procedure.

The day before the scheduled radiosurgery, the mask was placed in a 70°C water bath. After drying and cooling briefly, with a test for the patient's tolerable temperature, the mask was positioned and gently molded to the contours of the face. The mask was molded the day before so that it would dry completely.

A localizer was mounted on the mask system, serving as a reference for the acquisition of angiography and tomography scans. This localizer contains two copper squares and defines a precise three-dimensional stereotactic coordinate system within the patient's cranial volume. For localization, it was necessary to acquire a sagittal and a coronal image, with the two copper squares of the localizer completely visible in both images.

The patients then underwent computed tomography scans of the skull, carried out using a *multislice* device and iodinated contrast at a volume of 1 ml/kg.

After the CT scan, they underwent digital subtraction angiography in the hemodynamics room, using a *Philips Integris[1]* device, with pulsed fluoroscopy, digital images, *roadmapping*, *pixel shift*, using low-osmolarity iodinated contrast, in a total volume of approximately 100ml, injected by infusion pump. The angiography images, acquired in 2D, were acquired using fiducials to allow transfer and fusion with CT and MRI images, allowing delineation of the tissue (using images from all three exams simultaneously). Documentation was recorded in a digital file (report and images).

Finally, all the data (CT, MRI and angiography) was used in a computer program that allows image fusion, as well as the delineation of the organs at risk. Radiosurgery was planned using a collimator system with movable blades, associated with the BrainLab iPlan RT Image 4.1.1 and iPlan RT Dose 4.5.3 (Micro-Multileaf) planning systems[2] . The doses were determined based on the volume of the AVM and its topography, always trying to administer a dose of around 20 Gy in the periphery of the lesion when it was considered safe. Patients were treated on the 80% isodose curve for a single isocenter. Only non-embolized portions of AVMs were considered as targets for radiosurgery.

Radiosurgery itself was finally carried out using a Varian[3] 6MV linear accelerator.

4.6   Statistical analysis

The continuous quantitative variables were analyzed descriptively, with calculations of mean, standard deviation and median.

Student's t-test for two independent samples was used to compare the means of the study groups (such as the nidal volume and the prescribed dose), which were considered Gaussian (normal) by the Central Limit Theorem.

The Mann-Whitney non-parametric test was used for ordinal qualitative variables (samples with non-

1 Philips Medical System, Best, The Netherlands
2 rainLab, Munich, Germany
3 Varian, Inc., Palo Alto, California, USA

normal distribution, such as number of vessels and RBAS scale), making it possible to compare the median between two independent samples.

The bivariate chi-squared test (χ^2) was used to assess the association between categorical variables (such as topography, presence of arteriovenous fistula) and the outcome (cure), allowing comparisons between proportions.

The Kaplan-Meier test was used to verify the difference in healing time between patients grouped according to the type of intervention (radiosurgery alone or embolization followed by radiosurgery).

The significance level adopted was 5%.

5 RESULTS

5.1 Clinical, demographic and radiological data

This study included patients treated between July 2008 and December 2012 (allowing for 3-year post-treatment controls until December 2015). During this period, 61 patients with AVMs were treated by radiosurgery. We excluded 7 patients who underwent subsequent surgery (microsurgical resection of the lesion) and 7 patients without any post-radiosurgery follow-up data.

This study included 47 patients who underwent radiosurgery: 29 men (61.7%) and 18 women (38.3%). The mean age was 29.1 years, the maximum 70, and the minimum 7, with a median of 26 and a standard deviation of 15.1).

As for the initial clinical conditions, the patients were classified according to the modified Rankim scale (MRS, Appendix E). The radiological presentation of the AVM allowed classification according to the RBAS and modified Spetzler-Martin scales (both discussed in the literature review).

Table 1 summarizes the demographic data, initial clinical picture and radiological characteristics of the case.

Table 1 - Patient characteristics in terms of age, gender, volume (in ml), nidal topography, RBAS scale, initial presentation, pre-surgery MS and mRS grades.

Patient (RGHC)	Age	Sex	Liquid volume	Topography	RBAS	Presentation	SM	mRS
13738964I	50	M	4,9	Front	1,49	Headache	2	1
2244668H	30	M	13,5	Talamo	2,45	Bleeding	4	3
13743189E	40	M	6,4	Occipital	1,44	Bleeding	4	2
3286209J	26	F	0,5	Temporal	0,57	Bleeding	3B	1
3097100D	30	M	14,6	Parietal	2,06	Convulsion	4	1
88502975E	12	M	8,8	Talamo	1,62	Bleeding	4	2
5276451G	35	M	3,8	Talamo	1,58	Hypoesthesia	3B	1

continues

continuation

Patient (RGHC)	Age	Sex	Liquid volume	Topography	RBAS	Presentation	SM	mRS
13848574I	22	M	2,1	Temporal	0,65	Bleeding	3B	1
3354606C	19	M	1,9	Periventricular	0,57	Bleeding	3B	2
13777648F	46	M	3,3	Midbrain	1,75	Bleeding	3B	0
77079905C	30	F	0,6	Corpus callosum	0,66	Bleeding	3A	2
55430505J	21	M	1,1	Tàlamo	1,03	Bleeding	3B	0
13851011B	16	F	17,2	Corpus callosum	2,04	Bleeding	3A	0
13797863E	33	F	4,1	Front	1,07	Convulsion	2	0
55417544I	39	M	7,2	Front	1,50	Bleeding	3B	2
55425999J	14	M	20,7	Corpus callosum	2,35	Conv/cef	5	0
55720016K	34	F	3,8	Temporal	1,06	Bleeding	3A	0
88503129J	7	M	3,6	Periventricular	0,50	Bleeding	2	0
88503168J	70	F	0,2	NNBB	1,92	Bleeding	3B	3
13894594D	18	F	0,7	Midbrain	0,93	Bleeding	3B	2
13858924B	55	F	2,6	Front	1,36	Bleeding	3A	2

Patient (RGHC)	Age	Sex	Liquid volume	Topography	RBAS	Presentation	SM	mRS
88503251E	27	F	9,5	Front	1,49	Bleeding	3A	0
13765550G	14	M	3,4	Periventricular	0,62	Bleeding	3B	0
13894187I	8	M	0,5	Occipital	0,21	Bleeding	2	0
88504441F	63	M	1,8	Midbrain	1,94	Bleeding	3B	3
13875053	16	M	3,0	Tàlamo	1,12	Headache	4	0
88506227	9	M	3,9	Temporal	0,57	Hemiparesis	3B	2
13943911J	47	F	2,4	NNBB	1,68	Bleeding	3B	2
771052051	24	M	7,5	Front	1,23	Convulsion	5	1
13955777K	28	M	8,2	Front	1,38	Convulsion	4	0
13686784I	34	F	8,5	Cerebellum	1,53	Headache	2	0
88506664	45	F	8,0	Front	1,70	Bleeding	3A	2
88506424J	16	F	1,2	Front	0,44	Bleeding	2	2
88506478B	25	F	1,1	Parietal	0,61	Conv/cef	2	0
13853078K	15	F	3,4	Temporal	0,64	Conv/cef	4	0
13974478D	26	M	1,2	Temporal	0,64	Bleeding	3B	2
88506652	25	M	0,5	Tàlamo	1,05	Bleeding	3B	2
13792892	13	M	0,7	Tàlamo	0,83	Bleeding	3B	1
13986381G	16	M	0,5	NNBB	0,87	Bleeding	3A	1
13965625	24	M	1,2	Parietal	0,60	Headache	3B	0
13732630	61	M	1,1	Occipital	1,33	Bleeding	3B	1

Continued

Conclusion

Patient (RGHC)	Age	Sex	Liquid volume	Topography	RBAS	Presentation	SM	mRS
13995171	50	M	3,4	Cerebellum	1,34	Bleeding	2	3
88506690	34	F	7,5	Parietal	1,43	Bleeding	3A	0
13916458	20	F	1,8	Parietal	0,58	Bleeding	2	0
88506627	24	F	2,4	Front	0,72	Bleeding	3B	0
88506651G	27	M	1,3	Temporal	0,67	Headache	2	0
5292142G	34	M	1,5	Parietal	0,83	Hypoesthesia	2	1

Conv/cef: epileptic seizures and headache

mRS: modified Rankim scale[140]

NNBB: grassroots hubs

RBAS: Pollock-Flickinger scale ("Radiosurgery-based AVM Score")[84]

RGHC: patient's medical record number at the FMUSP Hospital das Clinicas. MS: modified Spetzler-Martin scale[2]

As for topography, 10 AVMs were in the frontal lobe (21.3%), 7 (14.8%) were in the temporal lobe, 7 (14.8%) were thalamic, and 6 (12.8%) were parietal. The other locations are shown in Table 2.

Table 2 - Distribution of AVMs according to topography in 47 patients.

Topography of the AVM	N	%
Front	10	21,3
Tàlamo	7	14,8
Temporal	7	14,8
Parietal	6	12,8
Occipital	3	6,4
Base cores	3	6,4
Brainstem	3	6,4
Periventricular	3	6,4
Corpus callosum	3	6,4
Cerebellum	2	4,3
Total	47	100

The patients were classified according to the Spetzler-Martin scale modified by Oliveira[2], which assesses the surgical prognosis of AVMs, and the grades ranged from II to V (Table 3). No patient with grade I AVM was treated by radiosurgery and/or embolization. The majority of patients treated (57.45%) had grade III AVMs.

Table 3 - Distribution of AVMs according to the Spetzler-Martin scale modified by Oliveira in 47 patients.

Spetzler-Martin- Oliveira score	N	%
II	11	23,40
III A	8	17,02
III B	19	40,43
IV	7	14,89
V	2	4,26
Total	47	100

The predominant initial symptoms were headaches and focal neurological deficits, as well as epileptic seizures. Table 4 summarizes the symptoms and signs in the 47 patients.

Table 4 - Absolute and relative frequency of initial symptoms in 47 patients.

Symptomatology	N	%
Headache	13	27,66
Hemiparesis	13	27,66
Epileptic seizures	7	14,89
Epileptic seizures and headache	5	10,64
Hemianopsia	2	4,26
Hemi-hypoesthesia	2	4,26
Syncope	2	4,26
Cranial nerve palsy	1	2,13
Aphasia and hemiparesis	1	2,13
Ataxia and headache	1	2,13
Total	47	100

Hemorrhagic cerebrovascular accident (intraparenchymal hematoma, subarachnoid and/or intraventricular hemorrhage) was the initial clinical event in 32 AVMs (68.1%). The second most common form of presentation was isolated headache (10.64%). The others are described in Table 5.

Table 5 - Distribution of patients in absolute numbers (n) and percentages (%) with regard to hemorrhagic presentation and other forms of clinical presentation.

Clinical Presentation	n	%
Bleeding	32	68,09
Headache	5	10,64
Convulsion	4	8,51
Seizure and Headache	3	6,38
Hemi-hypoesthesia	2	4,26
Hemiparesis	1	2,13
Total	47	100

Magnetic resonance imaging follow-up was carried out regularly in all 47 patients. The minimum follow-up was 24 months, the maximum 72 months, the average 36.1 months and the median 36 months. In 22 patients (46.81%), the MRI was suggestive of a cure.

After the MRI was suggestive of AVM occlusion, the patients underwent control digital cerebral angiography. In 17 cases (36%), angiography was requested because the MRI showed only a residual AVM. Of these, angiography showed angiographic occlusion of the AVM in only 1 case.

Angiographic occlusion of the AVM was observed in 23 patients (48.94%); other angiographic results are shown in Table 6.

Table 6 - Distribution of patients in absolute numbers (n) and percentages (%) with regard to angiographic findings at the last control angiography (n=47).

Control angiography	n	%
Total occlusion	23	48,94
Partial occlusion	8	17,02
Subtotal occlusion	3	6,38
Minimum response	5	10,64
No control angiography	8	17,02
Total	47	100

5.2 AVM angioarchitecture and bleeding events

In addition to the nidus itself, other changes associated with AVM were observed, with arteriovenous fistula being the most frequent, occurring in 24 patients (51.1%), either in isolation or associated with other changes (Table 7).

Table 7 - Distribution of patients in absolute numbers (n) and percentages (%) regarding the presence of vascular alterations associated with AVM (n=47).

Vascular alteration	n	%
Arteriovenous fistula	24	51,1
Venous stenosis	10	21,3
Venous ectasia	12	25,5
Nidal aneurysm	2	4,2
Proximal aneurysm	1	2,1

Patients with bleeding AVMs had arteriovenous fistulas in 62.5% of cases. AVMs with venous alterations - ectasia or stenosis - presented as hemorrhage in 83.3 and 90% of cases, respectively. All patients with arterial aneurysms suffered intracranial hemorrhage (Table 8).

Table 8 - Distribution of patients in absolute numbers (n) and percentages (%) regarding the presence of vascular alterations associated with AVM and the occurrence or not of hemorrhage as the initial clinical picture (n=47).

Change	n	Hemorrhagic (n)	%	Non-haemorrhagic (n)	%
Arteriovenous fistula	24	15	62,5	9	37,5
Venous ectasia	12	10	83,3	2	16,6
Venous stenosis	10	9	90,0	1	10,0
Nidal aneurysm	2	2	100,0	0	0
Proximal aneurysm	1	1	100,0	0	0

Intracranial hemorrhage was the exclusive presentation in all AVMs located in the occipital lobe, basal ganglia, brainstem and periventricular region.

Location in the parietal lobe was less associated with hemorrhagic presentation, as shown in Table 9.

Table 9 - Absolute (n) and relative (%) distribution of patients according to AVM topography and the occurrence or not of bleeding as a form of presentation.

Topography of the AVM n (%)	Hemorrhagic (n)	%	Non-haemorrhagic (n)	%

Temporal	7 (14,8)	4	57,1	3	42,8
Talamo	7 (14,8)	5	71,4	2	28,5
Parietal	6 (12,8)	2	33,3	4	66,6
Front	6 (12,8)	4	66,6	2	33,3
Frontoparietal	4 (8,5)	3	75,0	1	25,0
Occipital	3 (6,4)	3	100,0	0	0
Base cores	3 (6,4)	3	100,0	0	0
Brainstem	3 (6,4)	3	100,0	0	0
Periventricular	3 (6,4)	3	100,0	0	0
Corpus callosum	3 (6,4)	2	66,6	1	33,3
Cerebellum	2 (4,3)	1	50,0	1	50,0
Total	47 (100)	33		14	

5.3 Embolization results

A total of 26 patients (55.3%) were embolized before radiosurgery, with one or more sessions on separate days, for a total of 62 embolizations. 21 patients (44.7%) were not embolized, according to H0.

Table 10 - Distribution of patients in absolute numbers (n) and percentages (%) regarding the embolization sessions they underwent (n=47).

Embolization sessions	N	%
0	21	44,68
1	6	12,77
2	8	17,02
3	10	21,28
5	2	4,26
Total	47	100

Embolization was effective in reducing the size of the AVM in 23 (88.5%) of 26 embolized patients. The reduction in size was between 1 and 2 centimeters, as shown in Table 11.

Table 11 - Distribution of patients in absolute numbers (n) and percentages (%) as to whether or not the diameter of the AVM was reduced after embolization (n=26).

Spetzler-Martin- Oliveira pre-embolization score	Reduction in diameter (in centimeters) after one or more embolization sessions		
	0	1	2
	n	n (%)	n (%)	n(%)
II	6	3 (50,0)	3 (50,0)	0
IIIA	11	0	3 (27,3)	8 (72,7)
IIIB	7	0	6 (85,7)	1 (14,3)
IV	1	0	0	1 (100)
V	1	0	1 (100)	0
Total	26	3	13	10

All intranidal aneurysms were embolized. Arteriovenous fistulas were reduced and, in cases where there was a risk of significant penetration of embolic material into the venous system (when venous drainage of the AVM appears almost simultaneously with arterial opacification), they were left unchanged.

Clinical complications attributed to embolization are described in Table 12. These complications were clinically significant in the 2 cases of hemiparesis and in 2 of the cases of hemorrhage (increase of 2 or more points on the modified Rankim scale).

Table 12 - Distribution of patients in absolute numbers (n) and percentages (%) regarding the occurrence of complications after embolization (n=26).

Embolization sessions	Complications	
	Bleeding	Hemiparesis
	n (%)	n (%)
1	0	0
2	2 (7,7)	1 (3,8)
3	1 (3,8)	1 (3,8)
4	0	0
5	0	0
Total	3 (11,5)	2 (7,7)

5.4 Radiosurgery results

5.4.1 Angiographic occlusion of AVMs

Of the 47 patients who underwent radiosurgery, 35 (74.47%) received a single dose and 12 (25.53%) received a fraction of the total dose over 5 consecutive days.

The maximum clinical and radiological follow-up was 72 months (median 39 months). The average follow-up time between radiosurgery and cerebral angiography showing cure of the AVM was 31.45 months (minimum 24 months, maximum 40 months, with a median of 30 months).

AVM occlusion was achieved in 23 patients (48.94%). For the 26 patients whose AVMs were treated with embolization and radiosurgery, the occlusion rate was 46.15% (12 patients cured). For the 21 patients with AVMs treated only with radiosurgery, the occlusion rate was 52.38% (11 patients cured). There was no statistical difference between the two groups (p=0.772).

Graph 1 shows AVM occlusion over time, comparing the two groups (radiosurgery with and without embolization).

Graph 1 - Kaplan-Meier curve of the degree of angiographic occlusion of the AVM as a function of time for patients undergoing embolization and radiosurgery (green), and only radiosurgery (blue) n=47.

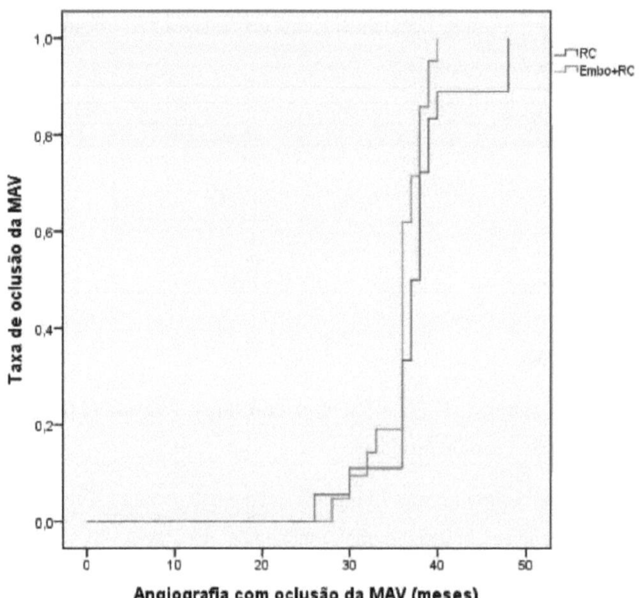

All AVMs reported as cured by MRI underwent cerebral angiography, which confirmed the occlusion. The average time between radiosurgery and angiography indicating occlusion was 36.04 months (minimum 26 months, maximum 48 months and median 37 months).

The univariate analysis of all the patients in the study showed that the volume of the nerve (p<0.001), the absence of an arteriovenous fistula at the time of radiosurgery (p=0.001), the prescribed dose (p=0.001) and a lower RBAS score (p=0.047) were significantly associated with AVM occlusion. Figure 4 shows the case of a patient with a bleeding left posterior parietal AVM with a RBAS of 0.83. Cure was achieved 3 years later after 1 embolization session followed by radiosurgery (1800Gy).

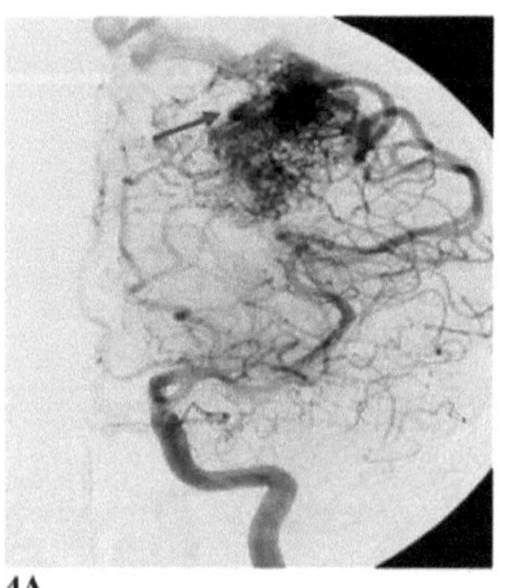

4A

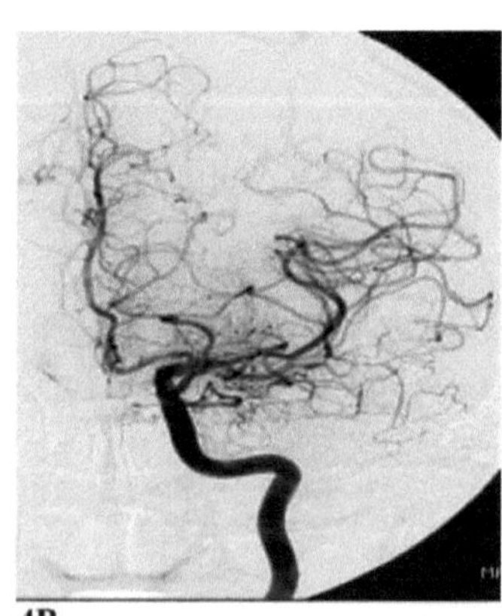

4B

Figure 4 - Left posterior parietal AVM (arrow) treated with embolization and radiosurgery in 2012 (A) with angiography in 2015 showing cure (B).

Regarding cure, there was no difference between superficial and deep AVMs, hemorrhagic presentation or not, restriction to venous drainage or not, deep or superficial venous drainage, presence of venous ectasia or not and previous embolization or not (according to the Chi Square test).

There was no difference between the median number of arteries in the groups of patients with and without angiographic cure (p=0.35), according to the Mann-Whitney test. Likewise, there was no difference between the number of veins in the groups of patients with and without angiographic cure (p=0.20), according to the same test.

The univariate analysis of the factors that may have contributed to the angiographic occlusion of AVMs is described in Table 13.

Table 13 - Distribution of patients in absolute numbers (n), with regard to mean, standard deviation (SD), median nidal volume, topography, RBAS scale, hemorrhagic presentation, number of nourishing arteries, presence or absence of arteriovenous fistula, number of draining veins, presence of venous drainage restriction, deep venous drainage, venous ectasia, previous embolization and prescribed dose, according to whether the AVM was occluded or not.

Variable	Healing	n	Average	dp	Median	p
nidal volume	Yes	23	2,66	2,22	1,80	**<0,001+**
	No	24	6,08	5,66	3,65	
topography (shallow vs. deep)	Yes	23				0,772J
	No	24				
RBAS scale	Yes	23	1,00	0,46	0,83	**0,047↑**
	No	24	1,31	0,59	1,37	
hemorrhagic presentation	Yes	23				0,680J
	No	24				
number of feeding arteries	Yes	23	2,52	0,59	3,00	0,350↑
	No	24	2,66	0,70	3,00	
arteriovenous fistula (absence vs. presence)	Yes	23				**0,001J**
	No	24				
number of drainage veins	Yes	23	1,65	0,64	2,00	0,205↑
	No	24	1,96	0,75	2,00	
presence of venous drainage restrictions	Yes	23				0,723J
	No	24				
presence of deep venous drainage	Yes	23				0,227J
	No	24				
presence of venous ectasia	yes	23				0,932J
	no	24				
prior embolization	yes	23	2,20	4,44	2,00	0,772J
	no	24				
prescribed dose cGy	yes	23	1,80	6,34	1,80	**0,001+**
	no	24				

+ Student's t-test; ↑ Mann-Whitney test; J $\chi2$ test

Lower nidal volume was associated with angiographic occlusion of the AVM ($p < 0.001$), as shown in Graph 2.

Graph 2 - *Box-plot* showing the differences in nidal volume between patients with angiographic occlusion of AVMs.

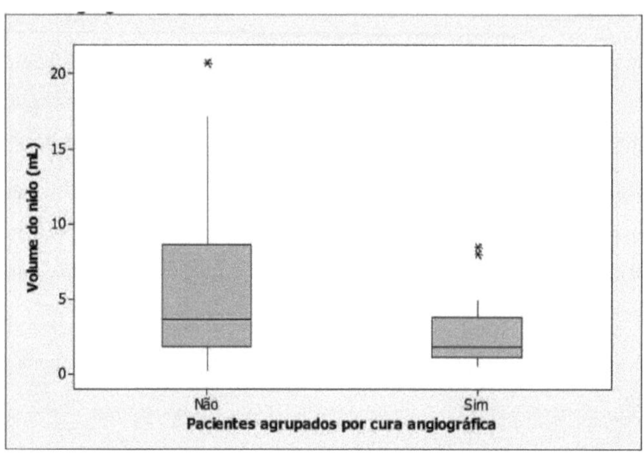

There was a significant difference (p=0.047) between the median scores on the RBAS scale of the groups of patients with and without angiographic cure: the lower the score, the greater the chance of cure, as shown in Graph 3.

Graph 3 - *Box-plot* showing the differences in degree on the RBAS scale between patients with angiographic occlusion of AVMs.

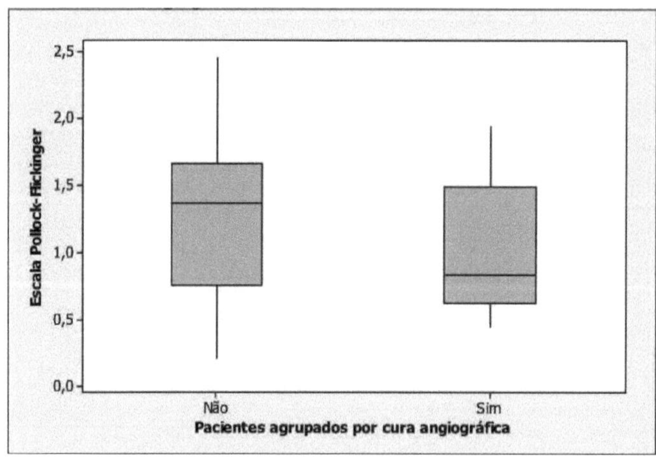

5.4.2 Favorable outcome of radiosurgery treatment

The favorable outcome (defined as angiographic occlusion of the AVM without the appearance of symptomatic radiation-induced changes and no post-treatment bleeding)[129] of the radiosurgery treatment was obtained in 19 patients (40.4%).

Clinical complications attributed to radiosurgery occurred in 4 of the total of 47 irradiated patients, as shown in Table 14. The two cases of hemorrhage were clinically significant (worsening of 2 points or more on the MRS), but did not require surgical treatment for hematoma drainage. Likewise, the two cases of radionecrosis (one of which is shown in Figure 5) had an increase of 2 points in the MRS, and were treated with corticosteroids, with stabilization of the condition.

Table 14 - Distribution of patients in absolute numbers (n) and percentages (%) regarding the occurrence of complications after radiosurgery (n=47).

Radiosurgery complications	n	%
Intracranial hemorrhage	2	4,3
Symptomatic radionecrosis	2	4,3
Total	4	8,5

The two cases of post-radiotherapy intracranial hemorrhage are worth detailing:

- One of the patients had undergone two prior embolization sessions (thalamic AVM with hemorrhagic presentation, nidal volume of 13.5cm^3 and RBAS of 2.45, presence of persistent intranidal AVF after embolization).

- The second was treated only with radiosurgery. Frontoparietal AVM, nidal volume of 7.5cm^3 and RBAS 1.23, initial presentation with epileptic seizures.

Both cases of radionecrosis:

- One of the patients (Figure 5) had a fronto-parietal AVM, a nidal volume of 14.6cm^3 and RBAS 2.06. Initial presentation with epileptic seizures. Not previously embolized. The last MRI scan showed a reduction in the nidus to 2cm^3.

- The second patient had a thalamic AVM (volume 3.8cm^3 and RBAS 1.58), clinical presentation with hemi-hypoesthesia (no bleeding), and underwent 3 embolization sessions. Despite an increase of 2 points in the mRS, he achieved angiographic cure in 40 weeks.

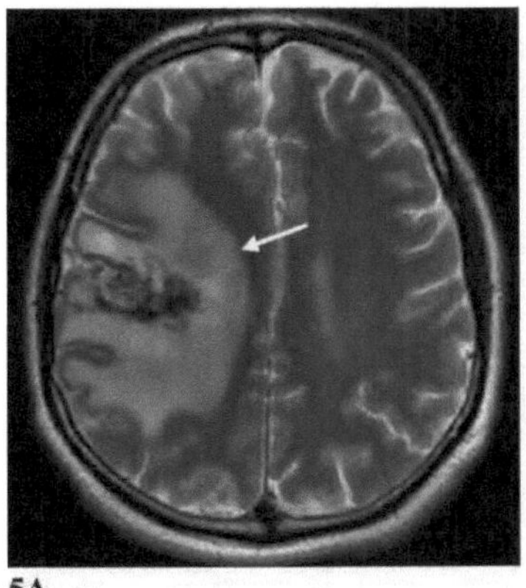

5A

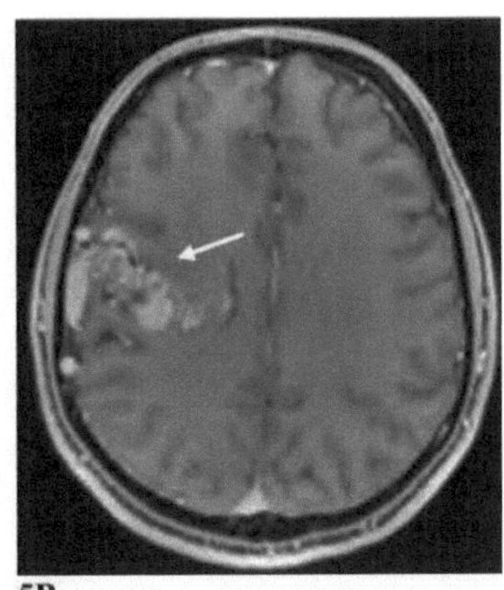

5B

Figure 5 - Radionecrosis - Area of signal alteration in T2 (arrow in A) surrounding the AVM node, in the right perirhinal region, with visible nidal enhancement (arrow in B). Multiple foci of hyposignal on T2 suggestive of hemosiderin (A).

Table 15 shows the distribution of the presence of an arteriovenous fistula within the AVM site and the favorable outcome. Figure 6 shows the case of a patient with a macrofistular component, irradiated in 2008, who presented with clinically significant bleeding in 2011.

Table 15 - Distribution of patients in absolute numbers regarding the presence of a fistula and whether or not a favorable outcome was obtained after radiosurgery (n=47).

Presence of AVF	Unfavorable result	Favorable result	Total
No	10	13	23
Yes	18	6	24
Total	28	19	47

p=0,051

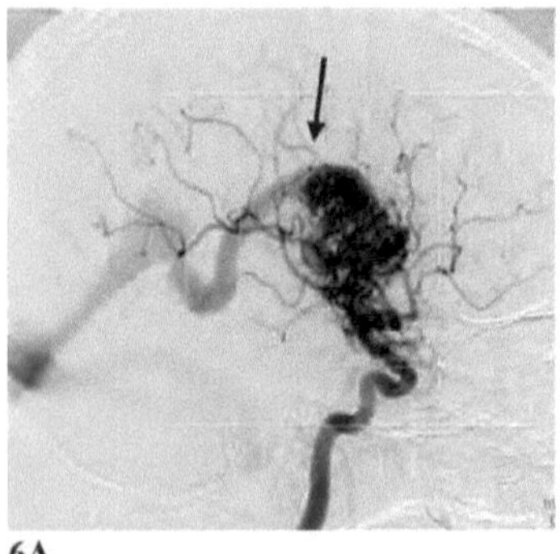

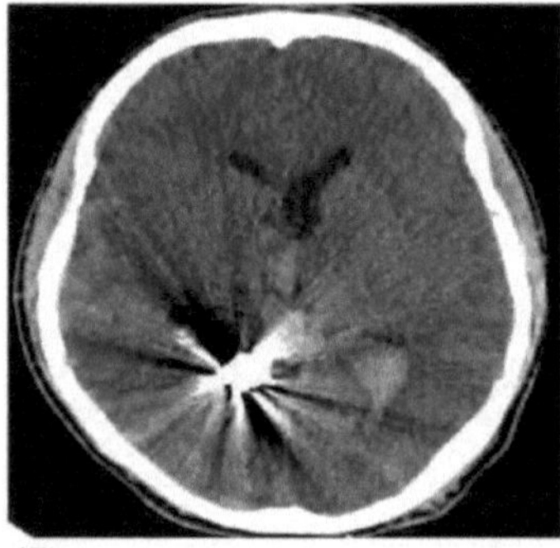

6A   6B

Figure 6 - AVM with macrofistular component (arrow), submitted to 2 embolization sessions. Undergoing radiosurgery (A), with a visible fistular component, she presented intracranial hemorrhage (B) 38 months later.

The hemorrhagic presentation of AVM occurred in 32 patients. There was no statistical correlation with the favorable outcome (p=0.558), as shown in Table 16.

Table 16 - Distribution of patients in absolute numbers with regard to the hemorrhagic presentation of AVM and whether or not a favorable outcome was obtained after radiosurgery

(n=47).

Hemorrhagic presentation	Unfavorable result	Favorable result	Total
No	8	7	15
Yes	20	12	32
Total	28	19	47

p=0,558

Applying a *cut-off* number equal to or less than 1 for the RBAS scale score, there was no association with a favorable result (p=0.172), as shown in Table 17.

Table 17 - Distribution of patients in absolute numbers according to the RBAS scale and whether or not a favorable outcome was obtained after radiosurgery (n=47).

RBAS less than 1	Unfavorable result	Favorable result	Total
No	19	8	27
Yes	9	11	20
Total	28	19	47

p=0,172

6 DISCUSSION

6.1 Patient selection, indications and post-treatment follow-up

AVMs are extremely heterogeneous lesions, with angioarchitecture and hemodynamics that vary between different patients and change over time. Combined therapy that includes embolization followed by radiosurgery is a minimally invasive method for AVMs that are difficult to treat due to the depth of the lesion, the morphological complexity and the high risk of definitive neurological damage with microsurgery[119].

In our series, the average nidal volume was 4.40ml (ranging from 0.24 to 20.70ml). The mean "radiosurgery-based classification of brain arteriovenous malformations" (RBAS) grade was 1.16 (ranging from 0.21 to 2.45), with a mode of 0.57 and a median of 1.07 (Table 1).

In the current literature, there is a tendency to irradiate large-volume AVMs ($> 10cm^3$), either by fractionating the dose (hypofractionated radiosurgery or repeating the treatment after a certain time interval) or by treating different geometric portions in several sessions, until the total volume of the lesion is reached. Both dose fractionation and volume fractionation aim to reduce radiation-induced radiological changes125,[129,141,142].

In our results, the topography of the AVMs (Table 2), as well as the indication for treatment based on the Spetzler-Martin scale, reflected what is in the literature[70, 143]: 58% of patients had grade 3 AVMs (Table 3). The same was true of the predominant symptomatology, the most frequent being the triad of headache, seizure and focal deficit[10] (Table 4).

In our study, a hemorrhagic cerebrovascular accident (intraparenchymal hematoma or subarachnoid hemorrhage) was the initial clinical event in 32 AVMs (68.1%), as shown in Table 5. Therefore, 15 (31.9%) non-routable AVMs were treated.

The criteria for whether or not to indicate therapeutic intervention for non-ruptured AVMs are not fully elucidated in the literature[24,25,144], with a strong tendency towards conservative treatment in the absence of evidence of hemorrhage. The only randomized study carried out to date[24] showed that the primary outcome, defined as symptomatic cerebrovascular accident or death, was observed in 10% of patients undergoing clinical treatment compared to 31% of those undergoing interventional treatment (microsurgery, radiosurgery or embolization, alone or in combination) (p<0.0001).

In our series, after the MRI suggested AVM occlusion, the patients underwent control digital cerebral angiography, as shown in Table 6. However, in 17 cases (36%), a control angiography was requested before the MRI suggested a cure, due to the longer time than 36 months after the radiotherapy treatment. In only one of these patients (in whom the MRI did not indicate a cure) was the angiographic finding that the AVM had been cured.

In a study of 140 patients[54], MRI correctly diagnosed 100% of patients who had total occlusion on angiography. The sensitivity of MRI seems to be related to the volume of the AVM[145]: volumes above 2.8cm^3 were the cut-off point above which the accuracy for predicting occlusion is over 90%. Despite the use of non-ionic contrast media, exams performed in high-volume centers[146] and more sophisticated equipment, cerebral angiography still has an incidence of 0.3 to 5.7% of neurological complications[147-149].

Routinely, post-treatment follow-up with digital subtraction angiography in all patients is unnecessary because the negative predictive value of post-radiosurgery MRI is high (> 90%)[62]. Evidence of AVM occlusion on MRI images was defined as the absence of "*flow-void*" on proton density, T1 and T2 weightings. Perineural contrast uptake was not taken into account, as this may not represent residual vessels, but localized breakdown of the blood-brain barrier caused by radiosurgery[150].

6.2   Changes in angioarchitecture and results

In our study, the vascular alterations associated with AVM found were, in order of frequency, intranidal arteriovenous fistula in 51.1% of cases, venous ectasia in 25.5%, venous stenosis in 21.3% and aneurysms in 6.3% of patients. In the case of venous stenosis, 90% of the cases in which it was present had a hemorrhagic presentation; all cases of AVMs with associated aneurysms, whether nidal or proximal, had hemorrhage as the initial presentation (Tables 7 and 8). These findings were also observed in the few articles that reported them[41,42].

The topography of hemorrhagic and non-hemorrhagic AVMs was relatively homogeneous, with a lower incidence of bleeding in parietal AVMs, but the study did not allow statistical analysis due to the small sample size (Table 9).

There was a statistically significant correlation between the presence of an arteriovenous fistula within the AVM node at the time of radiosurgery (also in patients who were embolized and persisted with AVF or in those who were not embolized) and a lower rate of angiographic occlusion (p=0.001).

When we consider not only the angiographic occlusion of the AVM, but also the absence of complications (hemorrhage or radionecrosis) related to the treatment, our study showed a strong correlation between the absence of AVF and favorable results. Although it didn't reach statistical significance of 5%, the presence of an arteriovenous fistula (AVF) within the AVM node seems to be a factor in failure (p=0.051). Eventually, a larger sample could lead to an association with statistical significance (Table 15).

In this regard, Meder *et al.*[81], considering Valavanis' definition[48], found that non-plexiform AVMs (those with AVF) had a low occlusion rate: only 1 in 13 AVMs (7.7%) were occluded by radiosurgery, compared to an occlusion rate of 75.3% in plexiform AVMs. Yuki *et al.*[104] demonstrated that embolization of only the fistular component is safe, due to a positive effect on reducing venous pressure, which would compensate for the increased flow to the AVM's nidal component. However, a study of AVMs such as ours, identifying fistulas within plexiform AVMs and demonstrating that they have a lower success rate than radiosurgery, had not yet been carried out.

In our study, there was no association between the presence of venous vascular alterations (number of draining veins, presence of restriction to venous drainage, presence of deep venous drainage, presence of venous ectasia) and the outcome of the treatment (Table 13), in agreement with the literature[62].

6.3   Results of radiosurgery and endovascular treatment

The 26 AVMs were embolized in one or more sessions using NBCA diluted in Lipiodol. Six patients (12.77%) received 1 session, 8 (17.02%) received 2 sessions, 10 (21.28%) 3 sessions and 2 patients (4.26%) received 5 embolization sessions.

Twenty-one patients (44.7%) underwent radiosurgery treatment without embolization (Table 10).

Embolization reduced the diameter of the AVM in 23 of the 26 patients embolized (88.5% effectiveness). In only 3 patients (all with grade II AVMs) was there no reduction in volume with embolization. In the others, the reduction in diameter (which reflects a reduction in AVM volume) ranged from 1 to 2 centimeters. In grade IIIA AVMs, this improvement reached 72.7% with a reduction of 2 centimeters (Table 11).

All intranidal aneurysms were embolized. Arteriovenous fistulas were reduced, but this lesion persisted in all cases; in cases where there was a risk of contrast penetrating the venous system, they were left unchanged. In the public health system, temporary flow reduction devices such as microballoons or *liquid coils* are not available, which makes it unsafe to attempt to embolize rapid arteriovenous fistulas (so-called macrofistulas, Figure 6).

Clinical complications attributed to embolization were defined as those occurring between embolization sessions and before the start of radiosurgery, and are described in Table 12. These complications occurred in 5 of the 26 embolized patients; of these, there were 3 cases (11.5%) of hemorrhage and 2 cases of focal neurological deficit (7.7%) attributed to ischemia.

The three cases of hemorrhage (confirmed by CT and MRI) were detected clinically in two patients by headache, followed by permanent motor deficit (increase of 2 points on the modified Rankim scale). In the third patient, a small cortical hemorrhage was clinically manifested by epileptic seizures, without deficits on neurological examination; this patient was fully controlled with anticonvulsant monotherapy. The morbidity rate reported in the literature[143,151,152] ranges from 3.8 to 30%, with a mortality rate of 1 to 3.7%.

In our series, the smaller volume of the nerve was associated with angiographic occlusion of the AVM (p<0.001), as was the prescribed dose (p=0.001). We observed a cluster of smaller AVMs among patients whose angiography showed occlusion of the lesion (Table 13 and Graph 2). In recent decades, the widespread use of linear accelerators and *"gamma knives"*, and the consequent evolution of planning *software*, planning with multiple superimposed images (MRI, CT and digital angiography) have provided a safer delineation of the lesion to be irradiated. The degree of occlusion (with consequent healing) of the AVM, without clinical complications, is related to the prescribed dose, which depends on the topography and volume treated[153].

Our results showed that there was no association between the hemorrhagic presentation of the AVM and angiographic occlusion, or with a favorable outcome (Tables 13 and 16), a finding that is at odds with the literature: for Ding *et al.*[138], hemorrhagic presentation of the AVM would have a beneficial impact on the response to radiosurgery, even in patients who were irradiated after complete resorption of the hematoma. In a multivariate analysis of 398 patients treated with radiosurgery, they found previous bleeding to be an independent factor in good response to radiosurgery (p=0.016). They hypothesized that the gliotic perineural capsule that develops after a hemorrhagic episode would facilitate the delineation of the nerve, which would become better defined radiologically.

Although the Spetzler-Martin scale has been developed and validated in numerous studies with the intention of evaluating the surgical prognosis of AVMs, it could also be correlated with the radiotherapy prognosis[88,154]. Even so, there are arguments that not all the elements of the scale are predictive of the final outcome[80] and that it does not correlate with the radiotherapy prognosis[81,82]. Other scales have therefore been developed with the aim of allowing a better correlation with the outcome of radiosurgery[83,84,88].

In our case, we evaluated one of these scales, the RBAS, which includes the patient's age, the volume of the AVM and the topography of the lesion. The grade ranged from 0.21 to 2.45. There was a favorable statistical correlation with angiographic healing of the lesion (p=0.047), as shown in Table 13 and Graph 3. However, in our sample, there was no association with a favorable outcome, assuming a *cutoff* equal to or less than 1 in the Chi-square test (p=0.172), as shown in Table 17.

Clinical complications attributed to radiosurgery were defined as those that occurred after the complete radiosurgery treatment. Such complications occurred in 4 of the total of 47 irradiated patients (Table 14).

In our study, intraparenchymal hemorrhages (confirmed by CT and MRI) in the latency period occurred in two patients (4.3%) and were detected clinically by headaches that were difficult to control, followed by neurological deficits (increase of 2 points on the modified Rankim scale), but there was no need to drain the hematomas; the neurological deficit remained unchanged until the last clinical check-up in both patients. The incidence of hemorrhagic stroke in the latency period reported in the literature[129,138] ranges from 2.3 to 17.8%.

Our results showed that radionecrosis was clinically manifested by seizures, hemiparesis and headache; the two cases (4.3%) responded well to corticosteroid therapy (symptoms stabilized). One of the patients in our series had a large (14.6cm^3) fronto-parietal AVM that had not previously been embolized. Radiosurgery was effective in reducing the nodule to 2cm^3, but with a persistent neurological deficit. The other patient (3.8cm thalamic AVM^3) was angiographically cured after 40 weeks, but also had a persistent neurological deficit. The incidence of radionecrosis described in the literature[152] is between 2.2 and 13%. Ironically, the appearance of hypersignal in T2 and FLAIR indicates a good prognosis after radiosurgery in terms of curing the AVM. However, when symptomatic, these same changes characterize radionecrosis[88].

Neodjuvant embolization is routinely used in up to 83% of radiosurgery series in the literature[102]. In our series, it was used in 55% of cases, with an effectiveness of 88.5% in what was proposed (volumetric reduction of the AVM).

Some studies[82,99,15]5 have shown that prior embolization would reduce the effectiveness of radiosurgery, as summarized above in the literature review. These studies did not take into account the protection provided by embolization against rebleeding during the latency period of radiosurgery. In our series, AVM occlusion was achieved in 46.15% of patients treated with embolization and radiosurgery, and in 52.38% of those treated with radiosurgery alone. There was no statistically significant difference (p=0.772) between the two groups, which can also be seen in the Kaplan-Meier curve (Graph 1). The evolution of endovascular techniques, with new materials[92], allowing flow interruption[93] for safer embolization, venous access[156], the use of double microcatheterization[157,158], are techniques that can bring greater safety and more consistent results, but are not available in our country's public health system.

This finding, when taken together with the finding that the presence of an arteriovenous fistula within the AVM seems to be a factor in its failure, suggests that neoadjuvant embolization (before radiosurgery) should have as its priority the elimination of the alterations associated with the AVM (AVFs and aneurysms) and not just the volumetric reduction of the lesion.

6.4 Limitations of this study

There were several limitations to this study, among them: it was a retrospective review with prospective follow-up, from a single center, which, because it is an uncommon disease, includes a relatively small number of patients and therefore has limited statistical power.

The clinical follow-up was not blinded, which increases the bias of the study and limits its external validity. AVMs of different sizes were grouped together and comparative analysis between the two scales (Spetzler-Martin and RBAS) was statistically unfeasible due to the small cohort.

Patients evaluated during the study period but not treated were not included, so there is no cohort or control group to define possible characteristics that could favor clinical treatment. All patients underwent treatment, and the decision to treat was certainly biased in relation to the clinical experience/opinion of the treating doctor.

Clinical and radiological follow-up after radiosurgery was limited (median 39 months, maximum 72 months); probably with longer follow-up, the degree of occlusion in some patients will be greater.

7 CONCLUSIONS

The absence of an intranidal arteriovenous fistula at the time of radiosurgery was the radiological alteration that showed a favorable statistical correlation with the cure (angiographic occlusion) of the AVM.

Venous alterations (ectasia, stenosis) present at the time of radiosurgery did not influence AVM healing.

The effectiveness (occlusion rate or radioanatomical cure) of the combined treatment (embolization + radiosurgery) was 46.15%.

The effectiveness (occlusion or radioanatomical cure rate) of treatment with radiosurgery alone was 52.38%.

There was no significant difference (p=0.772) between combined treatment (embolization + radiosurgery) and treatment with radiosurgery alone.

8 ANNEXES

8.1 Annex A - Informed Consent Form

HOSPITAL DAS CLiNICAS DA FACULDADE DE MEDICINA DA UNIVERSIDADE DE SAO PAULO TERMS OF FREE AND DISCLOSED CONSENT

IDENTIFICATION DATA OF THE RESEARCH SUBJECT OR LEGAL GUARDIAN

1   .PATIENT'S NAME: ....

IDENTITY DOCUMENT No :... SEX   : ▢ M F▢

DATE OF BIRTH: ..../......./......

ADDRESS .... APARTMENT APARTMENT: ....

NEIGHBORHOOD.. CITY ....STATE ....

ZIP CODE.. TELEPHONE: DDD(........)...........................

2   .LEGAL GUARDIAN ....

NATURE (degree of kinship, guardian, curator, etc.) ....

ID CARD : .... SEX: M F▢ ▢

DATE OF BIRTH..: ..../......./.....

ADDRESS .... APARTMENT APARTMENT: ....

NEIGHBORHOOD.. CITY ....STATE ....

ZIP CODE.. TELEPHONE:DDD(...........) ....

RESEARCH DATA

1. TITLE OF THE RESEARCH PROTOCOL: Evolutionary study of brain AVMs treated with radiosurgery previously submitted or not to embolization.

RESEARCHER: Dr. José Guilherme Mendes Pereira Caldas

POSITION: Full Professor

REGISTRATION REGIONAL COUNCIL OF MEDICINE No. 57.040

HCFMUSP UNIT: Institute of Radiology

3   . RESEARCH RISK ASSESSMENT:

▢ MINIMUM RISK▢ MEDIUM RISK▢ LOW RISK▢ HIGHER RISK

4   Duration of research: 4 years

HOSPITAL DAS CLiNICAS DA FACULDADE DE MEDICINA DA UNIVERSIDADE DE SAO PAULO (HCFMUSP) - RELEVANT INFORMATION.

1.   This information is being provided for your voluntary participation in this study. Arteriovenous malformations of the brain are rare diseases that are treated in various ways (surgery, embolization and radiosurgery) and the best way to control treatment results and prevent complications has yet to be determined.

2.   Procedures that will be used and purposes, including the identification of procedures that are experimental: There are no experimental procedures. All the tests to be carried out are routine, i.e. they would be carried out normally because of the illness, even if the patient were not part of the research.

Name of research subject or person responsible Name of researcher

3.   The main exams are

•   Cerebral angiography: performed under local anesthesia, catheter insertion into the femoral artery, injection of iodine-based contrast, exposure to X-rays for diagnosis.

•   Magnetic resonance imaging: performed without anesthesia, the patient lies down, without radiation, the device records the brain and the veins and arteries for diagnosis.

•   Tomography of the encephalon: performed without anesthesia, the patient lies down and radiation is used to register the brain for diagnosis.

4.   Expected discomforts and risks: Feeling unwell, nausea, allergic reaction to the contrast medium may occur. Low risk.

5.   There is no direct benefit for the research participant, only the fact that they are contributing to improving treatment and knowledge about this disease. The research aims to evaluate the effectiveness of treatment and early detection of possible complications. Only at the end of the study will we be able to conclude the presence of any benefits.

6.   Alternative procedures that may be advantageous for the patient to opt for: none.

7.   You are guaranteed the freedom to withdraw your consent to take part in this research at any time and to stop taking part in this study, without this causing any harm to your treatment and medical follow-up at HCFMUSP.

8.   Guaranteed access: at any stage of the study, you will have access to the professionals responsible for the research to clarify any doubts you may have.

9.   The principal investigator is Dr. Josè Guilherme Mendes Pereira Caldas, who can be reached at the institutional address and telephone number: Instituto de Radiologia do Hospital das Clinicas: Av. Dr. Enèas Carvalho de Aguiar 255.Phone: 3069-7086 or 3069-6389 or 3069-5492.

10.   If you have any considerations or questions about the ethics of the research, please contact the Research Ethics Committee (CEP) - Rua Ovidio Pires de Campos, 225 - 5o andar - tel: 2661-6442 ext. 16, 17, 18 - e-mail: .cappesq@hcnet.usp.br

Patient statement:

I have discussed my decision to take part in this study with Dr. Josè Guilherme Mendes Pereira Caldas. It was made clear what the objectives are, the procedures to be carried out, the risks, the guarantee of confidentiality and further clarification at any time. I know that my participation is completely voluntary, that I can withdraw at any time and that I am free of any expenses, and that I am guaranteed access to hospital treatment when necessary, in this health unit, whether or not I take part in this research.

Signature of patient or legal representative:____

Date: / ____/ ___

Signature of the person responsible for the study:____

Date: / ____/ ___

8.2 Annex B - Letter of Approval from the Department of Radiology and Oncology

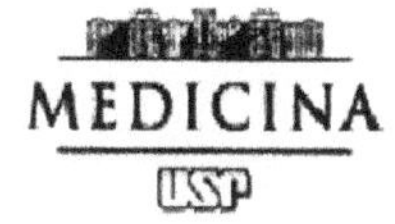

Departamento de Radiologia e Oncologia

Av. Dr. Arnaldo, 455, 455, 4° andar – sala 4123
CEP 01246-903
São Paulo - SP - Brasil
Fone/Fax: (11) 3061.7161

DRO - APROVAÇÃO 035/2013

APROVAÇÃO

O Departamento de Radiologia e Oncologia aprovou, em **06/06/2013**, o projeto de pesquisa:

Título do Estudo: "Estudo evolutivo das malformações arteriovenosas encefálicas tratadas com radiocirurgia, previamente submetidas ou não à embolização."

Pesquisador Responsável: José Guilherme Mendes Pereira Caldas
Pesquisador Executante: Carlos Michel Albuquerque Peres
Coordenador: Carlos Michel Albuquerque Peres

São Paulo, 05 de junho de 2013.

Prof. Dr. Manoel de Souza Rocha

**Profa. Dra. Maria Aparecida de Azevedo Koike Folgueira
Chefe do Departamento de Radiologia e Oncologia
FMUSP**

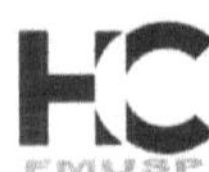

Hospital das Clínicas da FMUSP
Comissão de Ética para Análise de Projetos de Pesquisa - CAPPesq

PROJETO DE PESQUISA

Título: ESTUDO EVOLUTIVO DAS MALFORMAÇÕES ARTERIOVENOSAS ENCEFÁLICAS
TRATADAS COM RADIOCIRURGIA PREVIAMENTE SUBMETIDAS OU NÃO À EMBOLIZAÇÃO
Pesquisador Responsável: Jose Guilherme Mendes Pereira   **Versão: 2**
Caldas
Pesquisador Executante: Carlos Michel Albuquerque Peres   **CAAE:** 17627013.2.0000.0068
Co-autores: Evandro Cesar de Souza
Finalidade Acadêmica Doutorado
Instituição: HCFMUSP
Departamento: RADIOLOGIA E RADIOTERAPIA

PARECER CONSUBSTANCIADO DO CEP

Registro on-line: 11104

Número do Parecer: 522.359

Data da Relatoria: 05/02/2014

Apresentação do Projeto: Projeto bem apresentado, pertinente e de valor cientifico. Estudo retrospectivo e prospectivo de 30 pacientes tratados,com diagnostico de malformacao arteriovenosa dos vasos cerebrais, no periodo de 4 anos (de 2011 a 2014). Analise de series angiograficas, ressonancia magnetica e tomografia computadorizada pre e pos tratamento (endovascular e /ou radiocirurgia) de casos que evoluiram com complicacoes e dos nao complicados.

Objetivo da Pesquisa: Estudar a angioarquitetura das malformacoes arteriovenosas cerebrais, visando correlacionar alterações restritivas ao fluxo a ocorrencia ou nao de complicacoes precoces e tardias apos radiocirurgia ou no tratamento combinado com embolizacao.

Avaliação dos Riscos e Benefícios: O binomio riscos-beneficios e favoravel, considerando-se a gravidade das complicacoes e a importancia da avaliacao das caracteristicas arquiteturais das MAV em relacao ao prognostico da metodologia terapeutica.

Comentários e Considerações sobre a Pesquisa: A pesquisa esta bem elaborada, sendo analisados exames de diagnostico por imagem que fazem parte da avaliacao pre e pos operatorias rotineira das MAVs cerebrais. A descrição metodológica dos exames de imagem (angiografia, tomografia computadorizada e ressonancia magnetica) esta completa e detalhada, com estratificação do risco.

Considerações sobre os Termos de apresentação obrigatória: TCLE redigido de modo adequado e de acordo com a resolução 466 CONEP.

Recomendações: Nada a declarar.

Conclusões ou Pendências e Lista de Inadequações: Projeto aprovado.

Rua Dr. Ovídio Pires de Campos, 225 - Prédio da Administração - 5º andar
CEP 05403-010 - São Paulo - SP.
55 11 2661-7585 - 55 11 2661-6442 ramais: 16, 17, 18 | marcia.carvalho@hc.fm.usp.br

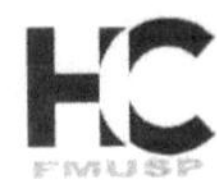

Hospital das Clínicas da FMUSP

Comissão de Ética para Análise de Projetos de Pesquisa - CAPPesq

Situação do Parecer: Aprovado

Necessita Apreciação da CONEP: Não.

Considerações Finais a critério do CEP: Em conformidade com a Resolução CNS nº 466/12 – cabe ao pesquisador: **a)** desenvolver o projeto conforme delineado; **b)** elaborar e apresentar relatórios parciais e final; **c)**apresentar dados solicitados pelo CEP, a qualquer momento; **d)** manter em arquivo sob sua guarda, por 5 anos da pesquisa, contendo fichas individuais e todos os demais documentos recomendados pelo CEP; **e)** encaminhar os resultados para publicação, com os devidos créditos aos pesquisadores associados e ao pessoal técnico participante do projeto; **f)** justificar perante ao CEP interrupção do projeto ou a não publicação dos resultados

São Paulo, 12 de Fevereiro de 2014

Prof. Dr. Alfredo José Mansur
-Coordenador
Comissão de Ética para Análise de
Projetos de Pequisa - CAPPesq

Rua Dr. Ovídio Pires de Campos, 225 - Prédio da Administração - 5º andar
CEP 05403-010 - São Paulo - SP.
55 11 2661-7585 - 55 11 2661-6442 ramais: 16, 17, 18 | marcia.carvalho@hc.fm.usp.br

8.4 Annex D - Clinical-Radiological Protocol

PROTOCOLO CLÍNICO-RADIOLÓGICOS DE DOENTES COM MALFORMAÇÕES
ARTERIOVENOSAS ENCEFÁLICAS SUBMETIDOS A RADIOCIRURGIA PRECEDIDA OU NÃO
DE EMBOLIZAÇÃO

Data da RC:__/__/__   Paciente:____
RGHC:____________   Registro PACS: _________ Sexo F M Idade__ Telefone:__________

Dados Clínicos	
Apresentação clínica	Cefaléia □ Crises convulsivas □ Hemiparesia □ Síncope □ Hemihipoestesia □ Hemianopsia □ Paralisia de nervo craniano □ Convulsão e cefaléia □ Ataxia □
Cirurgia prévia	Sim □ Não □
Escala de Rankim modificada pré-radiocirurgia	0 - Assintomático □ 1 - Sintomático mas independente □ Incapacidade: 2 - leve □ 3 - moderada □ 4- severa □ 5 - Acamado □ 6 - Óbito □
Escala de Rankim modificada 1 ano após a radiocirurgia	0 - Assintomático □ 1 - Sintomático mas independente □ Incapacidade: 2 - leve □ 3 - moderada □ 4- severa □ 5 - Acamado □ 6 - Óbito □

Ressonância Magnética	
Topografia: Frontal □ Temporal □ Parietal □ Occipital □ Tálamo □ Núcleos da base □ Periventricular □ Corpo caloso □ Cerebelo Mesencéfalo □	Diâmetro máximo do nido ___
Apresentação hemorrágica (RM inicial): Sim □ Não □	Ressonância intermediária ___ meses: Hemorragia □ Hipersinal em T2 perilesional □ Radionecrose □
Ressonância de controle final: Meses após radiocirurgia___ Hemorragia □ Hipersinal em T2 perilesional □ Radionecrose □	Cura □ Oclusão parcial □ Redução de volume □ Resíduo de MAV □ Inalterado (persistência da MAV) □

Angiografia cerebral digital	
Número de artérias _____	Fistula arteriovenosa Sim □ Não □
Aneurisma Proximal □ Distal □ Nidal □	Número de veias: _______
Estenose venosa Sim □ Não □	Drenagem venosa profunda Sim □ Não □
Ectasia venosa Sim □ Não □	Spetzler-Martin (usar diâmetro da RM):
Angiografia de controle final: _____ meses após radiocirurgia	Cura □ Oclusão subtotal □ Oclusão Parcial □ Resposta mínima □ Não tem angiografia de controle □

Embolização	
Número de sessões:	Agente embolizante:
Número de microcatéteres:	Microcateter(es) utilizado(s):
Redução de volume Sim □ Não □	Percentual aproximado de redução de volume: ___
Complicações Sim □ Não □	Especificar complicação:______________

Radiocirurgia		
Data: __/__/____	Dose prescrita:	Número de frações:
Dose mínima:	Dose máxima:	Isodose (%):

8.5   Annex E - Modified Rankim Scale

Modified Rankim Scale[131]

Pontos	Descrição
0	Assintomático / regressão dos sintomas
1	Sintomas não incapacitantes: consegue realizar tarefas habituais prévias.
2	Incapacidade leve: não consegue realizar todas as atividades habituais, mas capaz de realizar suas necessidades pessoais sem ajuda.
3	Incapacidade moderada: requer ajuda em tarefas habituais, mas consegue andar sozinho.
4	Incapacidade moderada a grave: não anda e precisa de ajuda para todas as atividades, inclusive pessoais.
5	Incapacidade grave: limitado ao leito, sem controle de esfíncteres, requer atenção constante.
6	Óbito

8.6 Annex F - Acceptance for publication in an indexed journal

Arquivos de Neuro-Psiquiatria

Decision Letter (ANP-2017-0108)

From: luisrmachado@globo.com

To: cmaperes@mac.com, cmaperes@usp.br

CC:

Subject: Arquivos de Neuro-Psiquiatria - Decision on Manuscript ID ANP-2017-0108

Body: 11-Apr-2017

Dear Dr. Peres:

It is a pleasure to accept your manuscript entitled "Brain arteriovenous malformations: The impact of associated nidal lesions in the outcome after radiosurgery alone or preceded by embolization. [Thesis]. São Paulo: "Faculdade de Medicina da Universidade de São Paulo"; 2017." in its current form for publication in the Arquivos de Neuro-Psiquiatria.

Thank you for your fine contribution. On behalf of the Editors of the Arquivos de Neuro-Psiquiatria, we look forward to your continued contributions to the Journal.

On July 1, 2015, SciELO will start to use a CC-BY license for all the publications in its collection. What does this mean?
All open-access systems need a license within the Creative Commons (CC) system so that they can operate without legal problems. The license most used within our setting (an also by Arquivos de Neuro-Psiquiatria) is the CC-BY-NC license, which presents some restrictions on how the information contained in the articles thus published is used. These restrictions are of a commercial nature: they do not apply to our journal, but they end up impairing its visibility in the open-access system.
The new CC-BY license ensures broader access to the articles published. SciELO has provided the following explanation:
" ... Among all the licenses, CC-BY is the one that is most effective for maximizing the dissemination of information, given that it is the least restrictive, provides a greater degree of freedom to reuse content and, like the other licenses, ensures that authorship is properly credited to the author or authors, and to the periodical or other means through which the article was originally published. This has the effect that the CC-BY license is the one that presents greatest compatibility when combined with other types of license, i.e. the content is released to fully interoperate with a wide variety of different systems and services, including commercial systems and services."

Sincerely,
Dr. Luis Machado
Editor-in-Chief, Arquivos de Neuro-Psiquiatria
luisrmachado@globo.com

Date Sent: 11-Apr-2017

Close Window

9 REFERENCES

1.   Spetzler RF, Martin NA. A proposed grading system for arteriovenous malformations. *J Neurosurg*. 1986;65:476-83.

2.   de Oliveira E, Tedeschi H, Raso J. Multidisciplinary approach to arteriovenous malformations. *Neurol Med Chir (Tokyo)*. 1998;38 Suppl:177-85.

3.   McCormick WF. The pathology of vascular ("arteriovenous") malformations. *J Neurosurg*. 1966;24:807-16.

4.   Atkinson RP, Awad IA, Batjer HH, Dowd CF, Furlan A, Giannotta SL, et al. Reporting terminology for brain arteriovenous malformation clinical and radiographic features for use in clinical trials. *Stroke*. 2001;32:1430-42.

5.   Al-Shahi R, Fang JS, Lewis SC, Warlow CP. Prevalence of adults with brain arteriovenous malformations: a community based study in Scotland using capture-recapture analysis. *J Neurol Neurosurg Psychiatry*. 2002;73:547-51.

6.   Al-Shahi R, Bhattacharya JJ, Currie DG, Papanastassiou V, Ritchie V, Roberts RC, et al. Prospective, population-based detection of intracranial vascular malformations in adults: the Scottish Intracranial Vascular Malformation Study (SIVMS). *Stroke*. 2003;34:1163-9.

7.   Fleetwood IG, Steinberg GK. Arteriovenous malformations. *Lancet*. 2002;359:863-73.

8.   Ruiz-Sandoval JL, Cantu C, Barinagarrementeria F. Intracerebral hemorrhage in young people: analysis of risk factors, location, causes, and prognosis. *Stroke*. 1999;30:537-41.

9.   Ogilvy CS, Stieg PE, Awad I, Brown RD Jr, Kondziolka D, Rosenwasser R, et al. Recommendations for the management of intracranial arteriovenous malformations: a statement for healthcare professionals from a special writing group of the Stroke Council, American Stroke Association. *Circulation*. 2001;103:2644-57.

10.   Abecassis IJ, Xu DS, Batjer HH, Bendok BR. Natural history of brain arteriovenous malformations: a systematic review. *Neurosurg Focus*. 2014;37:E7.

11.   Graf CJ, Perret GE, Torner JC. Bleeding from cerebral arteriovenous malformations as part of their natural history. *J Neurosurg*. 1983;58:331-7.

12.   Ondra SL, Troupp H, George ED, Schwab K. The natural history of symptomatic arteriovenous malformations of the brain: a 24-year follow-up assessment. *J Neurosurg*. 1990;73:387-91.

13.   Brown RD, Jr, Flemming KD, Meyer FB, Cloft HJ, Pollock BE, Link ML. Natural history, evaluation, and management of intracranial vascular malformations. *Mayo Clin Proc*. 2005;80:269-

81.

14.   Gross BA, Du R. Natural history of cerebral arteriovenous malformations: a meta-analysis. *J Neurosurg*. 2013;118:437-43.

15.   Forster DM, Steiner L, Hakanson S. Arteriovenous malformations of the brain. A long-term clinical study. *J Neurosurg*. 1972;37:562-70.

16.   Stefani MA, Porter PJ, terBrugge KG, Montanera W, Willinsky RA, Wallace MC. Angioarchitectural factors present in brain arteriovenous malformations associated with hemorrhagic presentation. *Stroke*. 2002;33:920-4.

17.   Brown RD, Jr, Wiebers DO, Torner JC, O'Fallon WM. Frequency of intracranial hemorrhage as a presenting symptom and subtype analysis: a population-based study of intracranial vascular malformations in Olmsted Country, Minnesota. *J Neurosurg*. 1996;85:29-32.

18.   Stapf C. Invasive treatment of unruptured brain arteriovenous malformations is experimental therapy. *Curr Opin Neurol*. 2006;19:63-8.

19.   Kondziolka D, McLaughlin MR, Kestle JR. Simple risk predictions for arteriovenous malformation hemorrhage. *Neurosurgery*. 1995;37:851-5.

20.   Brown RD, Jr. Simple risk predictions for arteriovenous malformation hemorrhage (correspondence). *Neurosurgery*. 2000;46:1024.

21.   Hernesniemi JA, Dashti R, Juvela S, Vaart K, Niemela M, Laakso A. Natural history of brain arteriovenous malformations: a long-term follow-up study of risk of hemorrhage in 238 patients. *Neurosurgery*. 2008;63:823-9;discussion 9-31.

22.   Stapf C, Mast H, Sciacca RR, Berenstein A, Nelson PK, Gobin YP, et al. The New York Islands AVM Study: design, study progress, and initial results. *Stroke*. 2003;34:e29-33.

23.   Stapf C, Mast H, Sciacca RR, Choi JH, Khaw AV, Connolly ES, et al. Predictors of hemorrhage in patients with untreated brain arteriovenous malformation. *Neurology*. 2006;66:1350-5.

24.   Mohr JP, Parides MK, Stapf C, Moquete E, Moy CS, Overbey JR, et al. Medical management with or without interventional therapy for unruptured brain arteriovenous malformations (ARUBA): a multicenter, non-blinded, randomized trial. *Lancet*. 2014;383:614-21.

25.   Amin-Hanjani S. ARUBA results are not applicable to all patients with arteriovenous malformation. *Stroke*. 2014;45:1539-40.

26.   Bharatha A, Faughnan ME, Kim H, Pourmohamad T, Krings T, Bayrak- Toydemir P, et al. Brain arteriovenous malformation multiplicity predicts the diagnosis of hereditary hemorrhagic

telangiectasia: quantitative assessment. *Stroke*. 2012;43:72-8.

27.   Komiyama M. Pathogenesis of brain arteriovenous malformations. *Neurol Med Chir (Tokyo)*. 2016;56:317-25.

28.   Komiyama M, Ishiguro T, Kitano S, Sakamoto H, Nakamura H. Serial antenatal sonographic observation of cerebral dural sinus malformation. *Am J Neuroradiol*. 2004;25:1446-8.

29.   Kim H, Su H, Weinsheimer S, Pawlikowska L, Young WL. Brain arteriovenous malformation pathogenesis: a response-to-injury paradigm. *Acta Neurochirurg Suppl*. 2011;111:83-92.

30.   Mahajan A, Manchandia TC, Gould G, Bulsara KR. De novo arteriovenous malformations: case report and review of the literature. *Neurosurg Rev*. 2010;33:115-9.

31.   Walker EJ, Su H, Shen F, Choi EJ, Oh SP, Chen G, et al. Arteriovenous malformation in the adult mouse brain resembling the human disease. *Ann Neurol*. 2011;69:954-62.

32.   Boudreau NJ, Varner JA. The homeobox transcription factor Hox D3 promotes integrin alpha5beta1 expression and function during angiogenesis. *J Biol Chem*. 2004;279:4862-8.

33.   Murphy PA, Kim TN, Lu G, Bollen AW, Schaffer CB, Wang RA. Notch4 normalization reduces blood vessel size in arteriovenous malformations. *Sci Transl Med*. 2012;4:117ra8.

34.   Morales-Valero SF, Bortolotti C, Sturiale C, Lanzino G. Are parenchymal AVMs congenital lesions? *Neurosurg Focus*. 2014;37:E2.

35.   Nussbaum ES, Heros RC, Madison MT, Awasthi D, Truwit CL. The pathogenesis of arteriovenous malformations: insights provided by a case of multiple arteriovenous malformations developing in relation to a developmental venous anomaly. *Neurosurgery*. 1998;43:347-51; discussion 51-2.

36.   Mouchtouris N, Jabbour PM, Starke RM, Hasan DM, Zanaty M, Theofanis T, et al. Biology of cerebral arteriovenous malformations with a focus on inflammation. *J Cereb Blood Flow Metab*. 2015;35:167-75.

37.   Sturiale CL, Puca A, Sebastiani P, Gatto I, Albanese A, Di Rocco C, et al. Single nucleotide polymorphisms associated with sporadic brain arteriovenous malformations: where do we stand? *Brain*. 2013;136:665-81.

38.   Hashimoto T, Wen G, Lawton MT, Boudreau NJ, Bollen AW, Yang GY, et al. Abnormal expression of matrix metalloproteinases and tissue inhibitors of metalloproteinases in brain arteriovenous malformations. *Stroke*. 2003;34:925- 31.

39.   Hashimoto T, Matsumoto MM, Li JF, Lawton MT, Young WL, University of California

SFBSG. Suppression of MMP-9 by doxycycline in brain arteriovenous malformations. *BMC Neurol.* 2005;5:1.

40.   Miyasaka K, Wolpert SM, Prager RJ. The association of cerebral aneurysms, infundibula, and intracranial arteriovenous malformations. *Stroke.* 1982;13:196-203.

41.   Redekop G, TerBrugge K, Montanera W, Willinsky R. Arterial aneurysms associated with cerebral arteriovenous malformations: classification, incidence, and risk of hemorrhage. *J Neurosurg.* 1998;89:539-46.

42.   Morgan MK, Alsahli K, Wiedmann M, Assaad NN, Heller GZ. Factors associated with proximal intracranial aneurysms to brain arteriovenous malformations: a prospective cohort study. *Neurosurgery.* 2016;78:787-92.

43.   D'Aliberti G, Talamonti G, Cenzato M, La Camera A, Debernardi A,

Valvassori L, et al. Arterial and venous aneurysms associated with arteriovenous malformations. *World Neurosurg.* 2015;83:188-96.

44.   Cagnazzo F, Brinjikji W, Lanzino G. Arterial aneurysms associated with arteriovenous malformations of the brain: classification, incidence, risk of hemorrhage, and treatment-a systematic review. *Acta Neurochir (Wien).* 2016.

45.   Mjoli N, Le Feuvre D, Taylor A. Bleeding source identification and treatment in brain arteriovenous malformations. *Interv Neuroradiol.* 2011;17:323-30.

46.   Clarencon F, Shotar E, Sourour NA. Comment on "Aneurysms Associated with Brain Arteriovenous Malformations". *Am J Neuroradiol.* 2017;38:E1-e4.

47.   Ramos Jr. FF, Nalli DR, Caldas JGMP. Endovascular Treatment of Cerebral Arteriovenous Malformations. In: Siqueira M, (ed.). *Tratado de Neurocirurgia.* Sao Paulo: EditoraManole; 2016. p. 739-56.

48.   Valavanis A, Pangalu A, Tanaka M. Endovascular treatment of cerebral arteriovenous malformations with emphasis on the curative role of embolization. *Interv Neuroradiol.* 2005;11:37-43.

49.   Han PP, Ponce FA, Spetzler RF. Intention-to-treat analysis of Spetzler-Martin grades IV and V arteriovenous malformations: natural history and treatment paradigm. *J Neurosurg.* 2003;98:3-7.

50.   Mast H, Mohr JP, Osipov A, Pile-Spellman J, Marshall RS, Lazar RM, et al. 'Steal' is an unestablished mechanism for the clinical presentation of cerebral arteriovenous malformations. *Stroke.* 1995;26:1215-20.

51. Spetzler RF, Hargraves RW, McCormick PW, Zabramski JM, Flom RA, Zimmerman RS. Relationship of perfusion pressure and size to risk of hemorrhage from arteriovenous malformations. *J Neurosurg.* 1992;76:918-23.

52. Laakso A, Hernesniemi J. Arteriovenous malformations: epidemiology and clinical presentation. *Neurosurg Clin N Am.* 2012;23:1-6.

53. Fullerton HJ, Achrol AS, Johnston SC, McCulloch CE, Higashida RT, Lawton MT, et al. Long-term hemorrhage risk in children versus adults with brain arteriovenous malformations. *Stroke.* 2005;36:2099-104.

54. Pollock BE, Flickinger JC, Lunsford LD, Bissonette DJ. Factors that predict the bleeding risk of cerebral arteriovenous malformations. *Stroke.* 1996;27:1- 6.

55. Cheng C-H, Crowley RW, Yen C-P, Schlesinger D, Shaffrey ME, Sheehan JP. Gamma Knife surgery for basal ganglia and thalamic arteriovenous malformations. *J Neurosurg.* 2012;116:899-908.

56. Mansmann U, Meisel J, Brock M, Rodesch G, Alvarez H, Lasjaunias P. Factors

associated with intracranial hemorrhage in cases of cerebral arteriovenous malformation. *Neurosurgery.* 2000;46:272-9- discussion 9-81.

57. Furlan AB, Figueiredo EG. Encephalic Arteriovenous Malformations. In: Figueiredo EG and Teixeira MJ, (eds.). *Manual de clinica neurocirùrgica.* Rio de Janeiro: Thieme Publicaçoes Ltda.; 2015. p. 26-31.

58. Amaro Jr. E, Ramos AO, Cardoso EF. Vascular diseases. In: Leite CC, Lucato LT and Amaro Jr. E, (eds.). *Neuroradiology: diagnostic imaging of brain changes.* Rio de Janeiro: Editora Guanabara-Koogan; 2011. p. 102-25.

59. Kucharczyk W, Lemme-Pleghos L, Uske A, Brant-Zawadzki M, Dooms G, Norman D. Intracranial vascular malformations: MR and CT imaging. *Radiology.* 1985;156:383-9.

60. Hadizadeh DR, von Falkenhausen M, Gieseke J, Meyer B, Urbach H, Hoogeveen R, et al. Cerebral arteriovenous malformation: Spetzler-Martin classification at subsecond-temporal-resolution four-dimensional MR angiography compared with that at DSA. *Radiology.* 2008;246:205-13.

61. Pollock BE, Flickinger JC, Patel AK, Bissonette DJ, Lunsford LD. Magnetic resonance imaging: an accurate method to evaluate arteriovenous malformations after stereotactic radiosurgery. *J Neurosurg.* 1996;85:1044-9.

62. Taeshineetanakul P, Krings T, Geibprasert S, Menezes R, Agid R, Terbrugge KG, et al. Angioarchitecture determines obliteration rate after radiosurgery in brain arteriovenous

malformations. *Neurosurgery*. 2012;71:1071-9.

63. Brown RD, Wiebers DO, Forbes G, O'Fallon WM, Piepgras DG, Marsh WR, et al. The natural history of unruptured intracranial arteriovenous malformations. *J Neurosurg*. 1988;68:352-7.

64. Pasqualin A, Barone G, Cioffi F, Rosta L, Scienza R, Da Pian R. The relevance of anatomic and hemodynamic factors to a classification of cerebral arteriovenous malformations. *Neurosurgery*. 1991;28:370-9.

65. Kothari RU, Brott T, Broderick JP, Barsan WG, Sauerbeck LR, Zuccarello M, et al. The ABCs of measuring intracerebral hemorrhage volumes. *Stroke*. 1996;27:1304-5.

66. Gobin YP, Laurent A, Merienne L, Schlienger M, Aymard A, Houdart E, et al. Treatment of brain arteriovenous malformations by embolization and radiosurgery. *J Neurosurg*. 1996;85:19-28.

67. Guo WY, Karlsson B, Ericson K, Lindqvist M. Even the smallest remnant of an AVM constitutes a risk of further bleeding. Case report. *Acta Neurochir*. 1993;121:212-5.

68. Sasaki T, Kurita H, Saito I, Kawamoto S, Nemoto S, Terahara A, et al. Arteriovenous malformations in the basal ganglia and thalamus: management and results in 101 cases. *J Neurosurg*. 1998;88:285-92.

69. Ellis TL, Friedman WA, Bova FJ, Kubilis PS, Buatti JM. Analysis of treatment failure after radiosurgery for arteriovenous malformations. *J Neurosurg*. 1998;89:104-10.

70. Starke RM, Komotar RJ, Hwang BY, Fischer LE, Otten ML, Merkow MB, et al. A comprehensive review of radiosurgery for cerebral arteriovenous malformations: outcomes, predictive factors, and grading scales. *Stereotact FunctNeurosurg*. 2008;86:191-9.

71. Miyamoto S, Hashimoto N, Nagata I, Nozaki K, Morimoto M, Taki W, et al. Posttreatment sequelae of palliatively treated cerebral arteriovenous malformations. *Neurosurgery*.2000; 46:589-94- discussion 94-5.

72. Raupp EF, Fernandes J. Does treatment with N-butyl cyanoacrylate embolization protect against hemorrhage in cerebral arteriovenous malformations? *Arq Neuropsiquiatr*. 2005;63:34-9.

73. Kader A, Goodrich JT, Sonstein WJ, Stein BM, Carmel PW and Michelsen WJ. Recurrent cerebral arteriovenous malformations after negative postoperative angiograms. *J Neurosurg*. 1996;85:14-8.

74. Morgan MK, Patel NJ, Simons M, Ritson EA, Heller GZ. Influence of the combination of patient age and deep venous drainage on brain arteriovenous malformation recurrence after surgery. *J Neurosurg*. 2012;117:934-41.

75. Sonstein WJ, Kader A, Michelsen WJ, Llena JF, Hirano A, Casper D. Expression of vascular endothelial growth factor in pediatric and adult cerebral arteriovenous malformations: an immunocytochemical study. *J Neurosurg.* 1996;85:838-45.

76. Lawton MT, Project UBAMS. Spetzler-Martin Grade III arteriovenous malformations: surgical results and a modification of the grading scale. *Neurosurgery.* 2003;52:740-8- discussion 8-9.

77. Heros RC, Korosue K, Diebold PM. Surgical excision of cerebral arteriovenous malformations: late results. *Neurosurgery.* 1990;26:570- 7;discussion 7-8.

78. Blackburn SL, Ashley WW, Rich KM, Simpson JR, Drzymala RE, Ray WZ, et al. Combined endovascular embolization and stereotactic radiosurgery in the treatment of large arteriovenous malformations. *J Neurosurg.* 2011;114:1758- 67.

79. Spetzler RF, Ponce FA. A 3-tier classification of cerebral arteriovenous malformations. Clinical article. *J Neurosurg.* 2011;114:842-9.

80. Hartmann A, Stapf C, Hofmeister C, Mohr JP, Sciacca RR, Stein BM, et al. Determinants of neurological outcome after surgery for brain arteriovenous malformation. *Stroke.* 2000;31:2361-4.

81. Meder JF, Oppenheim C, Blustajn J, Nataf F, Merienne L, Lefkoupolos D, et al. Cerebral arteriovenous malformations: the value of radiologic parameters in predicting response to radiosurgery. *Am J Neuroradiol.* 1997;18:1473-83.

82. Pollock BE, Flickinger JC, Lunsford LD, Maitz A, Kondziolka D. Factors associated with successful arteriovenous malformation radiosurgery. *Neurosurgery.* 1998;42:1239-44- discussion 44-7.

83. Pollock BE, Flickinger JC. A proposed radiosurgery-based grading system for arteriovenous malformations. *J Neurosurg.* 2002;96:79-85.

84. Pollock BE, Flickinger JC. Modification of the radiosurgery-based arteriovenous malformation grading system. *Neurosurgery.* 2008;63:239-43- discussion 43.

85. Burrow AM, Link MJ, Pollock BE. Is stereotactic radiosurgery the best treatment option for patients with a radiosurgery-based arteriovenous malformation score ≤ 1? *WorldNeurosurg.* 2014;82:1144-7.

86. Cohen-Inbar O, Ding D, Sheehan JP. Stereotactic radiosurgery for deep intracranial arteriovenous malformations, part 2: Basal ganglia and thalamus arteriovenous malformations. *J Clin Neurosci.* 2016;24:37-42.

87. Andrade-Souza YM, Zadeh G, Ramani M, Scora D, Tsao MN, Schwartz ML. Testing the radiosurgery-based arteriovenous malformation score and the modified Spetzler-Martin grading

system to predict radiosurgical outcome. *J Neurosurg*. 2005;103:642-8.

88.	Starke RM, Yen C-P, Ding D, Sheehan JP. A practical grading scale for predicting outcome after radiosurgery for arteriovenous malformations: analysis of 1012 treated patients. *J Neurosurg*. 2013;119:981-7.

89.	Missios S, Bekelis K, Al-Shyal G, Rasmussen PA, Barnett GH. Stereotactic radiosurgery of intracranial arteriovenous malformations and the use of the K index in determining treatment dose. *Neurosurg Focus*. 2014;37:E15.

90.	Sahlein DH, Mora P, Becske T, Nelson PK. Nidal embolization of brain arteriovenous malformations: rates of cure, partial embolization, and clinical outcome. *J Neurosurg*. 2012;117:65-77.

91.	Brassel F, Meila D. Evolution of embolic agents in interventional neuroradiology. *Clin Neuroradiol*. 2015;25 Suppl 2:333-9.

92.	de Castro-Afonso LH, Nakiri GS, Oliveira RS, Santos MV, Santos AC, Machado HR, et al. Curative embolization of pediatric intracranial arteriovenous malformations using Onyx: the role of new embolization techniques on patient outcomes. *Neuroradiology*. 2016;58:585-94.

93.	Chapot R, Stracke P, Velasco A, Nordmeyer H, Heddier M, Stauder M, et al. The pressure cooker technique for the treatment of brain AVMs. *J Neuroradiol*. 2014;41:87-91.

94.	Luessenhop AJ, Spence WT. Artificial embolization of cerebral arteries. Report of use in a case of arteriovenous malformation. *J Am Med Ass*. 1960;172:1153-5.

95.	Luessenhop AJ, Presper JH. Surgical embolization of cerebral arteriovenous malformations through internal carotid and vertebral arteries. Long-term results. *J Neurosurg*. 1975;42:443-51.

96.	Ding D, Sheehan JP, Starke RM, Durst CR, Raper DM, Conger JR, et al. Embolization of cerebral arteriovenous malformations with silk suture particles prior to stereotactic radiosurgery. *J Clin Neurosci*. 2015;22:1643-9.

97.	Yu SCH, Chan MSY, Lam JMK, Tam PHT, Poon WS. Complete obliteration of intracranial arteriovenous malformation with endovascular cyanoacrylate embolization: initial success and rate of permanent cure. *Am J Neuroradiol*. 2004;25:1139-43.

98.	Buell TJ, Ding D, Starke RM, Webster Crowley R, Liu KC. Embolization- induced angiogenesis in cerebral arteriovenous malformations. *J Clin Neurosci*. 2014;21:1866-71.

99.	Andrade-Souza YM, Ramani M, Scora D, Tsao MN, terBrugge K, Schwartz ML. Embolization before radiosurgery reduces the obliteration rate of arteriovenous malformations. *Neurosurgery*. 2007;60:443-51- discussion 512.

100. Xu F, Zhong J, Ray A, Manjila S, Bambakidis NC. Stereotactic radiosurgery with and without embolization for intracranial arteriovenous malformations: a systematic review and meta-analysis. *Neurosurg Focus*. 2014;37:E16.

101. Back AG, Vollmer D, Zeck O, Shkedy C, Shedden PM. Retrospective analysis of unstaged and staged Gamma Knife surgery with and without preceding embolization for the treatment of arteriovenous malformations. *J Neurosurg*. 2008;109 Suppl:57-64.

102. Izawa M, Chernov M, Hayashi M, Iseki H, Hori T, Takakura K. Combined management of intracranial arteriovenous malformations with embolization and gamma knife radiosurgery: comparative evaluation of the long-term results. *Surg Neurol*. 2009;71:43-52- discussion -3.

103. Bing F, Doucet R, Lacroix F, Bahary JP, Darsaut T, Roy D, et al. Liquid embolization material reduces the delivered radiation dose: clinical myth or reality? *Am J Neuroradiol*. 2012;33:320-2.

104. Yuki I, Kim RH, Duckwiler G, Jahan R, Tateshima S, Gonzalez N, et al. Treatment of brain arteriovenous malformations with high-flow arteriovenous fistulas: risk and complications associated with endovascular embolization in multimodality treatment. Clinical article. *J Neurosurg*. 2010;113:715-22.

105. Jayaraman MV, Marcellus ML, Hamilton S, Do HM, Campbell D, Chang SD, et al. Neurologic complications of arteriovenous malformation embolization using liquid embolic agents. *Am J Neuroradiol*. 2008;29:242-6.

106. Wikholm G, Lundqvist C, Svendsen P. The Goteborg cohort of embolized cerebral arteriovenous malformations: a 6-year follow-up. *Neurosurgery*. 2001;49:799-805- discussion -6.

107. Zabel du Bois A, Milker-Zabel S, Huber P, Schlegel W, Debus J. Risk of hemorrhage and obliteration rates of LINAC-based radiosurgery for cerebral arteriovenous malformations treated after prior partial embolization. *Int J Rad Oncol Biol Phys*. 2007;68:999-1003.

108. Barnett GH, Linskey ME, Adler JR, Cozzens JW, Friedman WA, Heilbrun MP, et al. Stereotactic radiosurgery--an organized neurosurgery-sanctioned definition. *J Neurosurg*. 2007;106:1-5.

109. Kano H, Kondziolka D, Flickinger JC, Yang HC, Flannery TJ, Niranjan A, et al. Stereotactic radiosurgery for arteriovenous malformations, Part 5: management of brainstem arteriovenous malformations. *J Neurosurg*. 2012;116:44-53.

110. Kano H, Kondziolka D, Flickinger JC, Yang HC, Flannery TJ, Niranjan A, et al. Stereotactic radiosurgery for arteriovenous malformations, Part 4: management of basal ganglia and thalamus arteriovenous malformations. *J Neurosurg*. 2012;116:33-43.

111. Betti OO, Munari C, Rosler R. Stereotactic radiosurgery with the linear accelerator: treatment of arteriovenous malformations. *Neurosurgery*. 1989;24:311-21.

112. Friedman WA. Stereotactic radiosurgery of intracranial arteriovenous malformations. *Neurosurg Clin N Am*. 2013;24:561-74.

113. Attia M, Menhel J, Alezra D, Pffefer R, Spiegelmann R. Radiosurgery-LINAC or gamma knife: 20 years of controversy revisited. *Israel Med Ass J*. 2005;7:583-8.

114. Schneider BF, Eberhard DA, Steiner LE. Histopathology of arteriovenous malformations after gamma knife radiosurgery. *J Neurosurg*. 1997;87:352-7.

115. Jahan R, Solberg TD, Lee D, Medin P, Tateshima S, Sayre J, et al. Stereotactic radiosurgery of the rete mirabile in swine: a longitudinal study of histopathological changes. *Neurosurgery*. 2006;58:551-8- discussion -8.

116. Picard L, Bollet MA, Anxionnat R, Bey P, Cordebar A, Jay N, et al. Efficacy and morbidity of arc-therapy radiosurgery for cerebral arteriovenous malformations: a comparison with the natural history. *Int J Rad Oncol Biol Phys*. 2004;58:1353-63.

117. Flickinger JC, Pollock BE, Kondziolka D, Lunsford LD. A dose-response analysis of arteriovenous malformation obliteration after radiosurgery. *Int J Rad Oncol Biol Phys*. 1996;36:873-9.

118. Inoue HK, Ohye C. Hemorrhage risks and obliteration rates of arteriovenous malformations after gamma knife radiosurgery. *J Neurosurg*. 2002;97:474-6.

119. Pollock BE, Gorman DA, Coffey RJ. Patient outcomes after arteriovenous malformation radiosurgical management: results based on a 5- to 14-year follow-up study. *Neurosurgery*. 2003;52:1291-6- discussion 6-7.

120. Friedman WA, Blatt DL, Bova FJ, Buatti JM, Mendenhall WM, Kubilis PS. The risk of hemorrhage after radiosurgery for arteriovenous malformations. *J Neurosurg*. 1996;84:912-9.

121. Pollock BE, Lunsford LD, Kondziolka D, Maitz A, Flickinger JC. Patient outcomes after stereotactic radiosurgery for "operable" arteriovenous malformations. *Neurosurgery*. 1994;35:1-7- discussion -8.

122. Maruyama K, Kawahara N, Shin M, Tago M, Kishimoto J, Kurita H, et al. The risk of hemorrhage after radiosurgery for cerebral arteriovenous malformations. *New Engl J Med*. 2005;352:146-53.

123. Chang JH, Chang JW, Park YG, Chung SS. Factors related to complete occlusion of arteriovenous malformations after gamma knife radiosurgery. *J Neurosurg*. 2000;93 Suppl 3:96-101.

124. Liscàk R, Vladyka V, Simonovà G, Urgosik D, Novotny J Jr, Janouskovà L, et al. Arteriovenous malformations after Leksell gamma knife radiosurgery: rate of obliteration and complications. *Neurosurgery*. 2007;60:1005-14- discussion 15-6.

125. Paùl L, Casasco A, Kusak ME, Martinez N, Rey G, Martinez R. Results for a series of 697 arteriovenous malformations treated by gamma knife: influence of angiographic features on the obliteration rate. *Neurosurgery*. 2014;75:568- 83- dicussion 82-3- quiz 83.

126. Lindqvist M, Karlsson B, Guo WY, Kihlstrom L, Lippitz B, Yamamoto M. Angiographic long-term follow-up data for arteriovenous malformations previously proven to be obliterated after gamma knife radiosurgery. *Neurosurgery*. 2000;46: 803-8- discussion 9-10.

127. Shin M, Kawamoto S, Kurita H, Tago M, Sasaki T, Morita A, et al. Retrospective analysis of a 10-year experience of stereotactic radio surgery for arteriovenous malformations in children and adolescents. *J Neurosurg*. 2002;97:779-84.

128. Blamek S, Tarnawski R, Miszczyk L. Linac-based stereotactic radiosurgery for brain arteriovenous malformations. *Clin Oncol*. 2011;23:525-31.

129. Moosa S, Chen CJ, Ding D, Lee CC, Chivukula S, Starke RM, et al. Volume- staged versus dose-staged radiosurgery outcomes for large intracranial arteriovenous malformations. *Neurosurg Focus*. 2014;37:E18.

130. Flickinger JC, Kondziolka D, Lunsford LD, Kassam A, Phuong LK, Liscak R, et al. Development of a model to predict permanent symptomatic postradiosurgery injury for arteriovenous malformation patients. Arteriovenous Malformation Radiosurgery Study Group. *Int J Rad Oncol Biol Phys*. 2000;46:1143-8.

131. Karlsson B, Jokura H, Yamamoto M, Soderman M, Lax I. Is repeated radiosurgery an alternative to staged radiosurgery for very large brain arteriovenous malformations? *J Neurosurg*. 2007;107:740-4.

132. Sirin S, Kondziolka D, Niranjan A, Flickinger JC, Maitz AH, Lunsford LD. Prospective staged volume radiosurgery for large arteriovenous malformations: indications and outcomes in otherwise untreatable patients. *Neurosurgery*. 2006; 58:17-27- discussion 17-27.

133. Souza EC. Results of radiosurgical treatment of patients with encephalic arteriovenous malformations classified as grades 3A, 3B, 4 or 5 previously submitted or not to embolization [Thesis]. *Faculty of Medicine*. Sao Paulo: University of Sao Paulo; 2010.

134. Mathis JA, Barr JD, Horton JA, Jungreis CA, Lunsford LD, Kondziolka DS, et al. The efficacy of particulate embolization combined with stereotactic radiosurgery for treatment of large

arteriovenous malformations of the brain. *Am J Neuroradiol.* 1995;16:299-306.

135. Miyachi S, Negoro M, Okamoto T, Kobayashi T, Kida Y, Tanaka T, et al. Embolization of cerebral arteriovenous malformations to assure successful subsequent radiosurgery. *J Clin Neurosci.* 2000;7 Suppl 1:82-5.

136. Samaniego EA, Kalousek V, Abdo G, Ortega-Gutierrez S. Preliminary experience with Precipitating Hydrophobic Injectable Liquid (PHIL) in treating cerebral AVMs. *J NeuroInterv Surg.* 2016:neurintsurg-2015-012210.

137. Vinuela F, Nombela L, Roach MR, Fox AJ, Pelz DM. Stenotic and occlusive disease of the venous drainage system of deep brain AVM's. *J Neurosurg.* 1985;63:180-4.

138. Ding D, Yen C-P, Starke RM, Xu Z, Sun X, Sheehan JP. Radiosurgery for Spetzler-Martin Grade III arteriovenous malformations. *J Neurosurg.* 2014;120:959-69.

139. Seldinger SI. Catheter replacement of the needle in percutaneous arteriography; a new technique. *Acta radiol.* 1953;39:368-76.

140. Farrell B, Godwin J, Richards S, Warlow C. The United Kingdom transient ischaemic attack (UK-TIA) aspirin trial: final results. *J Neurol Neurosurg Psychiatry.* 1991;54:1044-54.

141. AlKhalili K, Chalouhi N, Tjoumakaris S, Rosenwasser R, Jabbour P. Staged- volume radiosurgery for large arteriovenous malformations: a review. *Neurosurg Focus.* 2014;37:E20.

142. Abla AA, Rutledge WC, Seymour ZA, Guo D, Kim H, Gupta N, et al. A treatment paradigm for high-grade brain arteriovenous malformations: volume-staged radiosurgical downgrading followed by microsurgical resection. *J Neurosurg.* 2015;122:419-32.

143. Braksick SA, Fugate JE. Management of brain arteriovenous malformations. *Curr Treat Options Neurol.* 2015;17:358.

144. Cockroft KM, Jayaraman MV, Amin-Hanjani S, Derdeyn CP, McDougall CG, Wilson JA. A perfect storm: how a randomized trial of unruptured brain arteriovenous malformations' (ARUBA's) trial design challenges notions of external validity. *Stroke.* 2012;43:1979-81.

145. O'Connor TE, Friedman WA. Magnetic resonance imaging assessment of

cerebral arteriovenous malformation obliteration after stereotactic radiosurgery. *Neurosurgery.* 2013;73:761-6.

146. Thiex R, Norbash AM. Frerichs KU. The safety of dedicated-team catheterbased diagnostic cerebral angiography in the era of advanced noninvasive imaging. *Am J Neuroradiol.* 2010;31:230-4.

147. Earnest F, Forbes G, Sandok BA, Piepgras DG, Faust RJ, Ilstrup DM, et al. Complications of cerebral angiography: prospective assessment of risk. *Am J Roentgenol*. 1984;142:247-53.

148. Willinsky RA, Taylor SM, terBrugge K, Farb RI, Tomlinson G, Montanera W. Neurologic complications of cerebral angiography: prospective analysis of 2,899 procedures and review of the literature. *Radiology*. 2003;227:522-8.

149. Connors JJ, Sacks D, Furlan AJ, Selman WR, Russell EJ, Stieg PE, et al. Training, competency, and credentialing standards for diagnostic cervicocerebral angiography, carotid stenting, and cerebrovascular intervention: a joint statement from the American Academy of Neurology, the American Association of Neurological Surgeons, the American Society of Interventional and Therapeutic Neuroradiology, the American Society of Neuroradiology, the Congress of Neurological Surgeons, the AANS/CNS Cerebrovascular Section, and the Society of Interventional Radiology. *J Vasc Interv Radiol*. 2009;20:S292-301.

150. Parkhutik V, Lago A, Tembl JI, Vâzquez JF, Aparici F, Mainar E, et al. Postradiosurgery hemorrhage rates of arteriovenous malformations of the brain: influencing factors and evolution with time. *Stroke*. 2012;43:1247-52.

151. Hartmann A, Pile-Spellman J, Stapf C, Sciacca RR, Faulstich A, Mohr JP, et al. Risk of endovascular treatment of brain arteriovenous malformations. *Stroke*. 2002;33:1816-20.

152. Plasencia AR, Santillan A. Embolization and radiosurgery for arteriovenous malformations. *Surg Neurol Int*. 2012;3:S90-S104.

153. Lunsford LD, Kondziolka D, Flickinger JC, Bissonette DJ, Jungreis CA, Maitz AH, et al. Stereotactic radiosurgery for arteriovenous malformations of the brain. *J Neurosurg*. 1991;75:512-24.

154. Ding D, Yen C-P, Xu Z, Starke RM, Sheehan JP. Radiosurgery for patients with unruptured intracranial arteriovenous malformations. *J Neurosurg*. 2013;118:958-66.

155. Kano H, Kondziolka D, Flickinger JC, Park KJ, Iyer A, Yang HC, et al. Stereotactic radiosurgery for arteriovenous malformations after embolization: a case-control study. *J Neurosurg*. 2012;117:265-75.

156. Mendes GA, Iosif C, Silveira EP, Waihrich E, Saleme S, Mounayer C. Transvenous embolization in pediatric plexiform arteriovenous malformations. *Neurosurgery*. 2016;78:458-65.

157. Abud DG, Abud TG, Nakiri GS. Management of brain AVM procedural hemorrhagic complication by the "security" catheter technique. *J Neuroradiol*. 2013;40:45-9.

158. Abud DG, Riva R, Nakiri GS, Padovani F, Khawaldeh M, Mounayer C. Treatment of brain

arteriovenous malformations by double arterial catheterization with simultaneous injection of Onyx: retrospective series of 17 patients. *Am J Neuroradiol*. 2011;32:152-8.

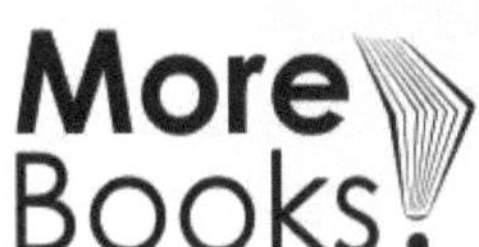

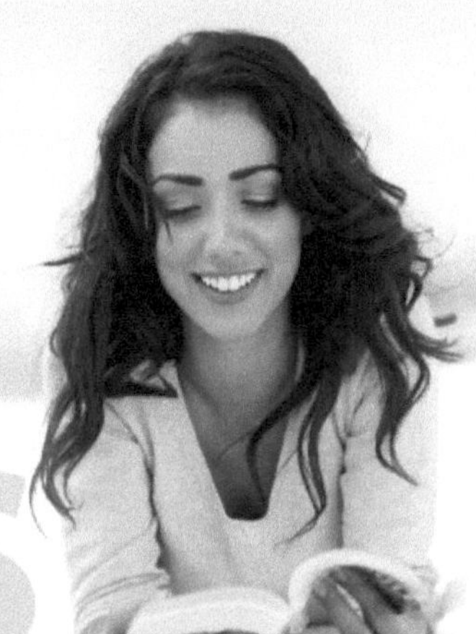

Buy your books fast and straightforward online - at one of world's fastest growing online book stores! Environmentally sound due to Print-on-Demand technologies.

Buy your books online at
www.morebooks.shop

Kaufen Sie Ihre Bücher schnell und unkompliziert online – auf einer der am schnellsten wachsenden Buchhandelsplattformen weltweit! Dank Print-On-Demand umwelt- und ressourcenschonend produzi ert.

Bücher schneller online kaufen
www.morebooks.shop

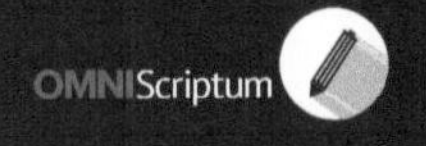

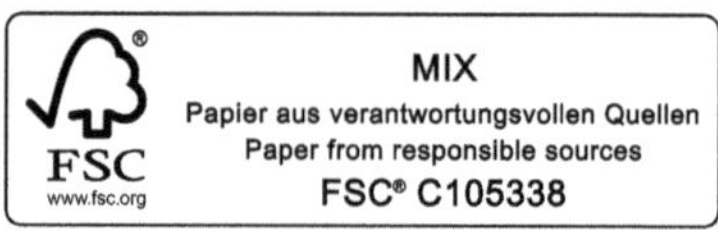

Printed by Books on Demand GmbH, Norderstedt / Germany